WHY YOU
REALLY HURT

IT ALL STARTS IN THE FOOT

D0958199

WHY YOU REALLY HURT

IT ALL STARTS IN THE FOOT

Dr. Burton S. Schuler

Why You Really Hurt: It All Starts in the Foot

Copyright 2009
By Dr. Burton S. Schuler
First Edition
Published by The La Luz Press, Inc.,
2001 W. 29th Street, Panama City, Fl 32405
(877) 698-6372, www.thelaluzpress.com

ISBN: 978-0-942664-02-7
LCCN: 2008907603

Publisher's Cataloging-In-Publication Data
(Prepared by The Donohue Group, Inc.)

Schuler, Burton S. (Burton Silverman), 1950-
Why you really hurt: it all starts in the foot / Burton S. Schuler.
p. : ill. ; cm.

Describes the discovery and treatment of Morton's Toe, named for Dr. Dudley J. Morton. Morton's Toe is an abnormality of the first metatarsal bone that the author contends is the basis of most foot problems, fibromyalgia, arthritis, and other body aches and pains. Also discusses the contributions of Dr. Janet Travell, White House physician during the Kennedy and Johnson administrations. Includes bibliographical references and index.

ISBN: 978-0-942664-02-7

1. Toes—Abnormalities—Treatment. 2. Chronic pain—Treatment. 3 Foot—Care and hygiene. 4. Morton, Dudley J. (Dudley Joy), b. 1884. 5. Travell, Janet G., 1901- I. Title.
RD786 .S38 2009
617/.585   2008907603

Designed by Rachelle Painchaud-Nash
Book Cover by Phil Velikan
Printed in Canada

*To my patients, the wonderful people of
Panama City, Bay County, and Northwest Florida,
who for the past twenty five years have allowed me
the daily joy of hopeful making them feel better,
and making them laugh.*

Acknowledgement

W hen I finally decided to sit down and get serious about writing this book, I had no idea that it would take me where it did and would introduce me to the wonderful group of people that it has. The following people made this book possible.

I'm indebted to the staff at the *John F. Kennedy Presidential Library* and *Museum of Boston*. I especially wish to thank Stephen Plotkin, Reference Archivist, who spent a great deal of time helping me hunt down the June, 1961 note that Robert F. Kennedy wrote about Dr. Travell. In addition, Cynthia Walker of the reference room was very helpful in locating a specific photo of President Kennedy and Dr. Travell I craved. Lyle Slovick, Assistant University Archivist, and G. David Anderson, University Archivist at the Gellman Library, George Washington University in Washington D.C., assisted me in regard to Dr. Travell's papers and collection. At the Lyndon B. Johnson Library and Museum in Austin, Ms. Morgan Blue was of great assistance to me. Laurie Langland, University Archivist at the George McGovern Library of Dakota Wesleyan University was very patient with me when I was looking for RFK's handwritten note to George McGovern. The staff at the Cushing/Whitney Medical Library, at the Yale University Medical School, and the medical library at Columbia University's College of Physicians and Surgeons were of great help to me.

My deepest thanks goes to Janice Berger, Sandy Morton, and Chris Morton, the grandchildren of Dudley Morton, who were very gracious with their time in telling me about their grandfather. I also thank them for sharing (for the first time with any researcher) the private letters, papers, and photos of him—that was invaluable to me in writing this book. My thanks also goes to Mrs. Virginia P. Street, daughter of Dr. Travell, who was always available when I had a question about her famous mother. My gratitude is offered to Dr. David Simons for taking the time to speak to me. Dr. Ben Daitz worked with Dr. Travell on the 1990 videotape, and I want to thank him for telling me all about how it was made.

I need to thank the folks at Columbia University Press, especially Sarah Scott, for giving me the clearance to reproduce Chapters 22 and 23 of *The Human Foot* in the appendix. Ms. Florence Eichen of the Penguin Group (USA) assisted me in getting printed the cover of Dr. Travell's autobiography. Thanks to my friends, the staff at the new and improved Bay County (Florida) Public Library for always getting me the books I requested and the research I needed. To the folks at the Cardinal Publishers Group, the Friesen Group and the La Luz Press, Inc., I appreciate your time and effect on my behalf.

At one time or another, several people worked on this book and helped to edit it. I need to thank them—this includes Joan Peace, Kate Estes and Connie Zales. But in the end it was Douglas Zang of Hawaii who did the bulk of the editing when I was wrapping up the book.

The one person who spent the most time on this book besides me was Rachelle Painchaud-Nash of Oakbank, Manitoba (that's in Canada). For about eighteen months, she has worked with me on numerous design changes to the book. I might have written every word but she is the one who got it down on paper. Thanks Rachelle.

The cartoon on page 22 was done by Kevin Goddu and was taken from my first book *The Agony of De-Feet*. Many of the photos, diagrams and drawing were done by Victor Strickland of beautiful Wewachitcha, Florida.

Again, thanks to all of you.

Introduction

Millions of people get out of bed hurting. Millions go through the day hurting. And millions more try to get a good sleep while hurting. I wrote this book for those people. If you are one of them or know someone who is, please believe me when I tell you there is hope in getting better. This hope is not based on pills, injections, surgeries, dietary supplements or arch supports. This hope is based on the work of two brilliant doctors and on well-established proven medicine that was first written about over eighty years ago, that I have seen help thousands of people. The hope is also based on using a simple little pad that goes on the bottom of your foot that you can make yourself for less than two dollars. For the past four decades, I have used this simple little pad to treat my patients to feel better, walk better, sleep better, and have less pain all over their body. If you follow my directions, there is a good chance that you can start feeling better at once.

Because of this, I know there is encouragement for many of you who believe that you might have to suffer forever with your aches and pains. It is highly unlikely that any doctor you have ever gone to has considered a very common foot condition known as Morton's Toe as the real reason for your suffering. This is not your doctor's fault. Despite the fact that Morton's Toe and the pains it could cause were well-known in the 1920s through 1950s, the modern physician was neither trained nor taught to recognize the torment it can cause. So it does not matter what you have been told in the past about why you hurt. It does not matter what tests, treatments or medications you have had. It does not matter that you may be even thinking about having surgery for your foot, knee, hip, leg, or back problem. The only thing that does matter is to find out if you do have a Morton's Toe and if any of your foot or body pains can get any better by just putting the simple pad on the bottom of your foot. Until you do that, you may never know if the real reason for your hurting is due to a Morton's Toe.

This is not a medical textbook. It was written for the average person. However, the book does have a bibliography and many endnotes throughout which support and document all of the long-established medicine and other facts that I have presented. I know some of the medical terms and words that I use in the book may be confusing. So for that reason, I have also included a glossary. If you find a word that has a ★ next to it (e.g., Joint★), you can find the meaning of that word starting on page 191 of the appendix.

Even though this book is about medical conditions, I wrote it so it would be easy to read and simple to understand. I hope I have achieved that goal.

Burton S. Schuler, D.P.M., D.A.A.P.M.
Panama City, FL

Contents

Chapter 6

Chapter 7

Chapter 8

Chapter 9

Chapter 10

Chapter 11

Dry Bones

The foot bone connected to the leg bone,
The leg bone connected to the knee bone,
The knee bone connected to the thigh bone,
The thigh bone connected to the back bone,
The back bone connected to the neck bone,
The neck bone connected to the head bone,

AUTHOR UNKNOWN

Part 1

Chapter 1

The Best $8.00 I Ever Spent

One day, during my sophomore year at the New York College of Podiatric Medicine, I stopped by the little bookstore on the top floor of the school. In my free time, I would often go there to check out the new books that arrived. That day, I was looking around and noticed a stack of books I had never seen before. On the very bottom of that stack was an older book that appeared to have been there for some time. It was more worn, dusty and beaten up than the newer books, and undoubtedly had seen better days. As I read the title, I had no idea as to the importance this book would represent in my future. The book was entitled *The Human Foot* by Dr. Dudley J. Morton, and was published in 1935 by the Columbia University Press.[1] Since I was planning to spend my professional life as a foot specialist, I thought that price allowing, it might not be a bad idea to own a book called *The Human Foot*. I asked the clerk, "How much for the book?" After checking numerous lists and catalogs, he was unable to find a price for it. In frustration, he said to me, "Look, the cheapest book in the store is $8.00, so you can have it for that."

Now, you must understand that $8.00 was a lot of money to me in 1972. It would have paid for two movie tickets and a pizza, which back then, was a really hot date for me and my then girlfriend. So I had a major choice:

1

hot date or a book by some guy named Dudley. It was a close call, but I took Dudley home with me that night, and my girlfriend had to settle for a tuna fish sandwich, no movie, and the simple pleasure of my company (she had a wonderful time). Thirty-five years later, I cannot even remember the girl's name or what she looked like, but to this day, I use what I learned in that one book and because of it, I have helped a lot of people.

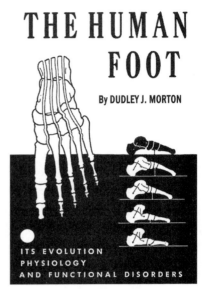

Fig. 1-1. Book cover of the The Human Foot, *written by Dudley J. Morton, M.D., First published in 1935 by Columbia University Press (courtesy Columbia University Press).*

Good News

I hope you find this book easy to read and understand. It is all about one single bone in your foot, the first metatarsal bone, and whether the one you were born with is working correctly. If your first metatarsal bone is not working the way it should be because the first bone is shorter than the second bone, then you may have a common foot condition known as Morton's Toe (Fig. 1-2). Morton's Toe is not a new medical condition. In fact, it was first written about 80 years ago[2].

It has been well established by several admired medical doctors that the Morton's Toe is a major cause of aches, pains and torment not only of the feet and ankles, but also of the back, hips, thighs, calves, knees, legs and

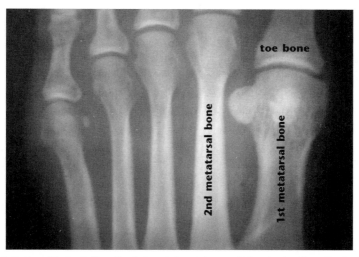

Fig. 1-2. In a Morton's Toe, the 1st metatarsal bone will be shorter than the 2nd metatarsal bone.

other places all over your body. It can even be a cause of fibromyalgia. I personally believe it can cause sleep disturbances and possibly be a contributing cause of Restless Legs Syndrome. The good news is that all of the pains and problems associated with Morton's Toe can by treated by putting one simple little inexpensive pad on the bottom of your foot or in your shoe. I am hoping that what you will read in the following pages will help you feel better.

What this Book Will Do for You

The aim of this book has always been to help get people out of pain as quickly as possible. In order to do this, I designed the book to be in two parts.

Part I is written so it would be as easy as possible to find in one place all the information on why you are really hurting and what to do about it quickly, easily, and cheaply.

By the end of Part I, you will hopefully:

- know what Morton's Toe is;

- know if you have a Morton's Toe;

- know if any aches or pains in your feet or body are caused by Morton's Toe;

- know how to make a simple pad for your foot or shoe, *for only two or three dollars,* that will treat the problems associated Morton's Toe; and

- learn about the lives of Dr. Dudley J. Morton and Dr. Janet Travell, the doctors who were associated with the concept of the Morton's Toe and with all of the problems it could cause.

Part II contains a lot of other important information, but it is not needed in getting you feeling better quickly. Part II contains information about:

- Myofascial pain, fibromyalgia and Morton's Toe;

- Diabetic ulcers, amputations, and the Morton's Toe;

- More about the life of Dr. Morton; and

- Why arch supports really don't work and the national ripoff associated with them.

There is also an appendix that contains a glossary and re-prints of Chapter 22 and 23 of Dr. Morton's book *The Human Foot,* and other interesting things.

Two Doctors

Two of the most noted physicians of the twentieth century were linked with defining the condition of the Morton's Toe and the pains and treatment associated with it. The most important physician in the story of the

Morton's Toe is Dr. Dudley J. Morton, the man whose name it bears. He was an orthopedic surgeon, who during his career, taught at both Yale and Columbia Medical Schools. In the 1920s he wrote two articles about the problems one can have by being born with abnormalities of the first metatarsal bone, or as it has come to be known, Morton's Toe. The articles were published in the highly respected *Journal of Bone and Joint Surgery,* the leading medical journal in its field[3]. For the next thirty years, Morton was recognized as one of the foremost medical experts in the world when it came to problems of the human foot and its treatments. I will tell you much more about Dudley J. Morton in Chapter 10 and how his work could help you.

The other physician who is essential to this story is Dr. Janet Travell. She was no ordinary doctor. From 1961-1965 she served as the personal White House physician to Presidents John F. Kennedy (Fig. 1-3) and Lyndon B. Johnson and their families[4], the first woman ever to do so. Robert F. Kennedy felt that Dr. Travell, in fact, changed the history of the United States by being partially responsible for making John F. Kennedy the thirty-fifth President of the United States[5].

She understood the importance of the Morton's Toe, or the "Dudley J. Morton Foot," as she called it. Dr. Travell knew that having a Morton's Toe could be the real cause of having pain from your head to your toes. This was because Morton's Toe could be one of the causes of a body-wide painful condition of the muscles called Myofascial Pain Syndrome. She knew what she was writing and talking about concerning Myofascial Pain Syndrome. You see, Dr. Janet Travell was and is still considered by many people to be the world's leading author-

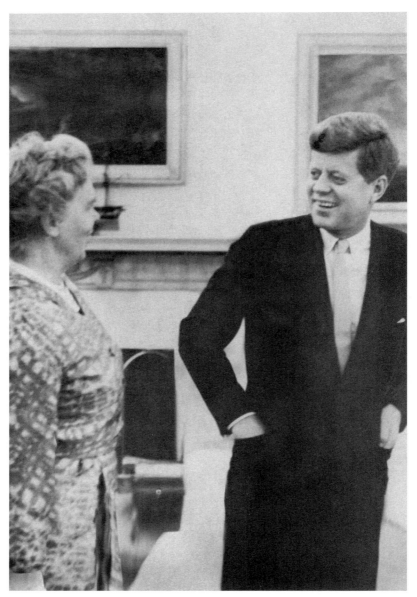

Fig. 1-3. President John F. Kennedy, with Dr. Janet Travell, his personal physician, in the White House, spring 1961 (John F. Kennedy Library).

ity on Myofascial Pain Syndrome. Her two-volume book, called *Myofascial Pain and Dysfunction: The Trigger Point Manual,* coauthored by Dr. David Simons, is still the leading authority on this painful body-wide medical problem[6]. For decades, she alerted the medical profession about the significance of Morton's Toe as being a cause of Myofascial Pain Syndrome. She was so dedicated to this mission that at the age of 89, she made a series of videotapes to teach the medical profession about Myofascial Pain Syndrome. One of these tapes was specifically made about the Morton's Toe in order to assist doctors in recognizing and treating it.[7] I will further discuss Dr. Travell, JFK, LBJ, RFK, Myofascial Pain Syndrome, trigger points and why your body may hurt all over, in Chapter 11. Trust me, it is a fascinating story.

Why and How I Wrote this Book

I had known for many years that the pain and suffering associated with having Morton's Toe was easily treatable with a simple pad on the bottom of the foot. And, it was based on good, proven medicine, developed by two eminent physicians: Dr. Morton and Dr. Travell. What I could not understand or accept was why this treatment, capable of relieving so much suffering, was not known or used by more doctors. Could it be that I was the only doctor who ever read *The Human Foot?*

During the last twenty-five years or so, it was rare to read anything in any medical or podiatric publication about the effects of having a Morton's Toe or about how to treat it. Nor was it lectured about at any medical meeting that I was aware of. Because of that, I became very frustrated. Knowing how important the work of Morton and Travell was in reducing pain, I knew I had to do something to re-introduce it to the public and medical profession. Sometime in the early 1990s, I toyed with the idea of writing a book about the Morton's Toe. To be honest, the idea of writing another book did not thrill me. My first book, *The Agony of De Feet, a Podiatrist Guide to Foot Care*[8], took a great deal of time to research and write, and the process was very demanding. I got lucky, and the book was very well received around the country. But after that book, I decided that birthing one book was enough for me, and I had no desire to write another one.

Never Say Never

So there I was in the early 1990s, not wanting to write another book, but knowing deep down inside that I really had to. Knowing that, I did what came naturally: I procrastinated. I always looked for, and found some excuses or distraction that got in the way of me writing this book. However, during those years, I kept telling everyone that I was writing a book about the Morton's Toe and its treatment. Eventually, my family, friends, patients and staff got so sick and tired of me running my mouth about the book that they told me to write the damn thing or shut up! So, by popular request, sometime around 2003–2004, I finally started to write. And ladies and gentlemen – here we are.

The people of this country spend billions and billions of dollars a year treating pain, be it pain medications prescribed by personal physicians, over-the-counter pain killers like aspirin or acetaminophen, creams or ointments, special shoes, arch supports, copper bracelets, back braces, special beds, Tens units, dietary supplements, or numerous other items. We will try almost anything to feel better. I hope that the day may come when we routinely look at our feet and decide if we really need any of the above or just a simple "toe pad" to feel better. The following pages will explain how and why this should and could be possible.

Chapter 2

What is a Morton's Toe?

On the next page, I will tell you, but first allow me to tell you a story. In June of 2006, I appeared on National Public Radio's *People's Pharmacy,* hosted by Teri and Joe Graedon. I was there to discuss Morton's Toe, its causes and why it could be the long-forgotten reason not only for your foot pain, but for also having pain throughout the entire body. One of the major causes for having a Morton's Toe is the abnormal condition when the first metatarsal bone is shorter than the second metatarsal bone (Fig. 2-1). Man, I really thought I was doing a wonderful job of explaining this until Joe Graedon reminded me, in a very diplomatic way, that I first needed to describe to the listeners what a metatarsal bone was, and where it was located in the foot. Because I deal with the metatarsal bones daily, I just assumed that everyone knew what they were and where they were located. Of course, I was

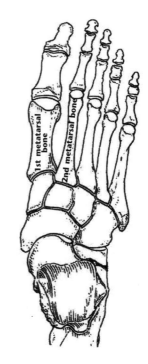

Fig 2-1. Skeleton of foot showing short first metatarsal bone and long second metatarsal bone.

wrong in this assumption! So, before we start, I need to explain to *you* what the metatarsal bones are and where they are located.

The five metatarsal bones are the finger-like bones to which the toes attach. They extend about halfway down your foot, toward your heel. They are inside your foot so you really cannot see them except for the bump that is down and outside of your big toe. This bump is the "head" of the first metatarsal bone. The only way to see the true length of the metatarsal bones is with an X-ray.

For the purpose of this book, and to make it as easy as possible for you to understand, "Morton's Toe" will mean having either one or both of two abnormal, inherited conditions of the first metatarsal bone of the foot.

The first abnormal condition, and the most noted one, that can cause Morton's Toe is when your first metatarsal bone is shorter than your second metatarsal bone.

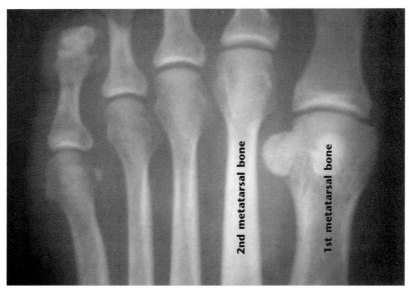

See how much shorter the first metatarsal bone is compared to the second metatarsal bone above. This is a Morton's Toe.

The second condition is when your first metatarsal bone is not as stable as it should be, and as a result, has too much motion. This is known as "Hypermobility of the First Metatarsal Bone."

Do You Have a Short First Metatarsal Bone?

Look down at your feet. Socks off please! If your second toe seems longer, (and I mean even just a hair longer) than your first toe, you may have a short first metatarsal bone.

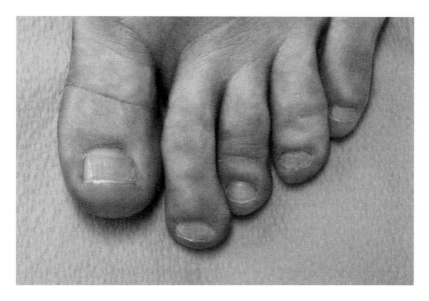

The above photograph shows a classic Morton's Toe caused by a short first metatarsal bone. Note how the big toe is shorter, and the second toe is longer and sticks out more. Morton's Toe is normally not this noticeable. Most of the time in a Morton's Toe, the big toe will appear to be only a little shorter than the second toe or just about the same length as the second toe.

Another way to check to see if you have a short first metatarsal bone is to hold your first and second toes down. Right behind the spot where the toes attach to the foot, you will see bumps pushing up from the top of your foot. These bumps are the heads of the first and second metatarsal bones. Using a pen, lipstick, or marker, draw a line where the bumps end (flat area) and meet the top of the foot. This spot is the very end of both of the heads of

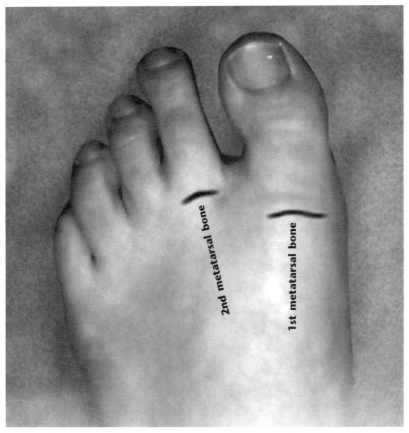

Fig. 2-2. See how the line at the 2nd metatarsal head is further down the foot than the line at the first metatarsal head. This means the first metatarsal bone is shorter than the 2nd metatarsal bone, and this person most probably has a Morton's Toe .

the first and second metatarsal bones. Look at both lines. If the line of the second metatarsal head is farther down your foot toward your toes than the first metatarsal head, even just a very little, then you probably have a short first metatarsal bone (Fig. 2-2).

Sometimes it is not necessary to draw a line on top of the foot because the relationship of the metatarsal heads can easily be seen. If this is the case, you can see without difficulty that the second metatarsal head is farther down the top of the foot than the first metatarsal head.

Frequently, people with short first metatarsal bones will also have a "webbing" between their second and third toes.[1] They will have a flap of excess skin that sort of looks like a "bat wing" in between the second and third toes (Fig. 2-3). If you do have this webbing of the toes, it is a pretty good tip off that you either have a short metatarsal bone or you are part duck. Check to see if Mom or Dad, or anyone else in the family has this also.

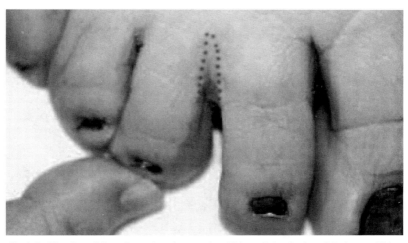

Fig 2-3. The dotted line show the abnormal webbing of the 2nd and 3rd toes. This is a indicator that this person does have a short first metatarsal bone.

Do You Have Hypermobility of the First Metatarsal Bone?

Unlike the short first metatarsal bone, there is no simple reliable way that you can determine on your own if you have hypermobility of the first metatarsal bone. But because it is treated the same way as the short first metatarsal bone, with the Toe Pad discussed in detail in Chapter 8, it is not that important for you to know for sure if you have hypermobility or not. What counts is if you feel any better once you start to treat yourself for your Morton's Toe.

Dr. Morton stated that there was a third possible reason for having a Morton's Toe besides a short or hypermobile first metatarsal bone.

There are two small bones that sit normally right under the head of the first metatarsal bone. They are

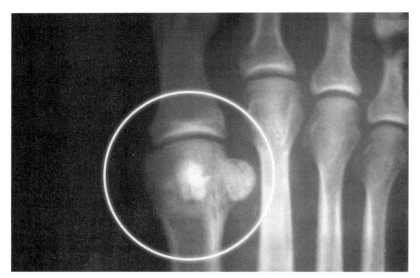

Fig. 2-4. Circled picture of two sesamoid bones under the head of the first metatarsal bone.

called the sesamoid bones (Fig. 2-4). If these bones, for whatever the reason, move backwards away from the head of the bone, it would make the first metatarsal bone meet the ground abnormally, in the same way a short first metatarsal bone would.

But Morton felt that the displaced sesamoid bones were a minor player in our foot problems, and did not seem to affect the foot to the same degree as the other two conditions did.[2]

Dr. Morton recognized that besides having either a short first metatarsal bone or hypermobility of that bone, there were many other actions, stresses, strains, and forces that affected the way your foot works and that can cause and contribute to foot problems. At no time or place did Dr. Morton ever state that having either of those conditions was a *guarantee* of having a foot problem or any other problem.[3] The only thing he ever stated was that having the short first metatarsal bone or hypermobility of the first metatarsal bone *may* lead to foot problems. This is very important and you need to be aware of it.

Why is this Important, or Pain from Head to Toe

For several years, many of the patients I was treating for their foot problems due to Morton's Toe were repeatedly telling me how much better they were feeling in other places on their bodies. They were happy because their feet were not only getting better, but also their backs, thighs, knees, legs and hips were also feeling better following my treatments. Many told me they were also sleeping better because of fewer leg cramps during the night. Some even told me their fibromyalgia was hurting less. I knew there was something special going on, but it did not immediately sink in. Heck, I was just happy their feet were doing better!

It was not until about the time I finished my certification to become a Diplomate of the American Academy of Pain Management that I finally realized what my patients had been trying to tell me for years—a Morton's Toe could also cause chronic pain almost anywhere in the body! I also finally "got it" because of the book published around that time by Drs. Janet Travell and David Simon on Myofascial Pain Syndrome. That book showed that Morton's Toe was one of the underlying causes of this extremely painful muscular condition that could cause pain all over.

Let me make this simple. Many of the following listed aches, pains and conditions not only of the feet but of the whole body may be caused by Myofascial Pain because you have either a short 1st metatarsal bone or hypermobility of the 1st metatarsal bone.[4]

- back pain
- hip pain
- knee pain
- leg pain
- plantar fasciitis
- calf pain
- fibromyalgia
- arthritis
- burning feet
- bunions
- fallen arches

- ankle pain
- heel pain
- arch pain
- weak ankles
- hammer toes
- tired feet (all over)
- neuromas
- corns and calluses
- shooting pains in the toes
- stress and march fractures
- night cramps (restless leg syndrome)
- temporo-mandibular joint pain (TMJ)
- diabetic foot ulcers

Doctors tell millions of people every day that the reason for their aches and pains is because they have "arthritis." But these doctors never explain to the patients **WHY** they have arthritis to start with. I believe that in many cases, Morton's Toe is the explanation for this **WHY**, and the reason for other pains in their back, knee, hip or lots of other places in their body.

So the bottom line is this: if your feet hurt and you do have a Morton's Toe, it may not be an accident that you ended up in the office of your local podiatrist or physician. Or that you have spent money on these problems with the result that no one, no medicine, or nothing, has been able to help.

The Toe Pad

If you are hurting and think you might have Morton's Toe, I will teach you how to treat it yourself. In Chapter 8, you will be shown how to make the simple Toe Pad, or Shoe Insert (Fig. 2-5). They will address the aches and pains of your feet and body that are associated with Morton's Toe. This pad, or shoe insole, has been working one way or another for over eighty years.[5] The Toe Pad is a patented, proven medical treatment, that has withstood the test of time. It is not a work in progress. It is not an arch support or a special shoe that costs hundreds of dollars and will not work. It is a simple pad or insole that can be made for about $2.00-$3.00 and will work better than any arch support can.

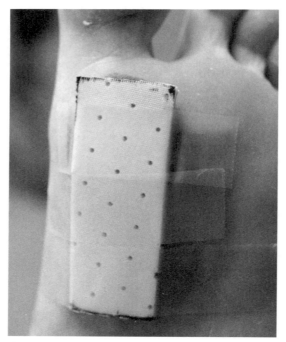

Fig. 2-5. This is the basic toe pad that goes under the first metatarsal bone which is the treatment for Morton's Toe.

Chapter 3

Do You Have a Morton's Toe or the Wrong Type of Inheritances?

Heredity is one of the major causes for having foot problems. When someone says that you look like your mom or dad, bear in mind that the resemblances can also extend to how your feet look and act. It is not unusual for me to examine three generations of one family only to see the Morton's Toe, or other similar foot problems, are present in all three generations. Most people think the reasons their feet are hurting are because of a bad pair of shoes, having the wrong job or just standing too much. I don't believe so. Don't misunderstand, those things (job, shoes, standing) can definitely aggravate a foot already susceptible to having problems, but by themselves, they are rarely the real underlying causes of the foot problems. They are simply the external stresses that finally push your feet over the edge in mid-life, causing you to have pain. When I tell patients for the first time that their foot problems are NOT likely due to their job, shoes, and/or standing on their feet too much, but rather due to Ma, Pa, or Uncle Louie, they look at me dumbfounded.[1] Think about it. Does everyone you work with, who has the same job as you, stand on the same floor for as long as you do, or wear the same exact style shoe as you, have foot problems? Of course not! Then why do you and not them? It is because in the great lottery of life, you were

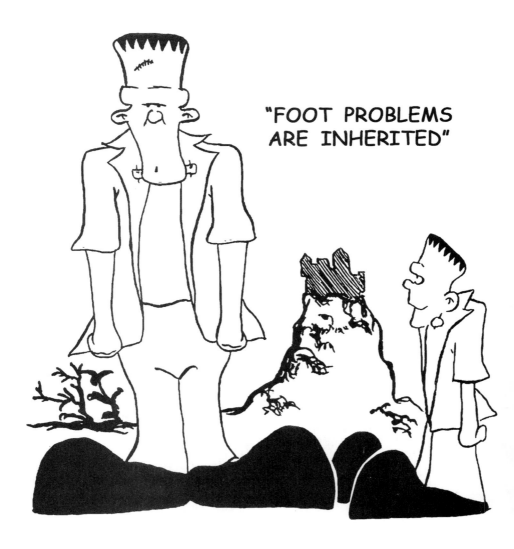

born with the tendency to have a Morton's Toe or some other foot problem. Of course, if you knowingly wear shoes that are wrong for your feet, they will hurt. In regard to shoes, don't forget that famous age old saying,

"You cannot fit a salami into a hot dog bun."

Patients ask me all the time, "Dr. Schuler, what can I do to prevent my foot problems?" My answer is simple:

"Pick different parents next time,
when it comes to your feet."

Most people who inherit the tendency to have foot problems don't have these problems until they reach middle age. That is when these inherited traits start to take their toll due to the day-in, day-out trauma that has built up over the years.

Dr. Morton explained this in his 1952 book, *Human Locomotion and Body Form.*[2] He stated that the tissues of the youthful foot have more elasticity than those of the older foot, and because of that, most foot problems do not appear until after thirty years of age. Morton went on to

Human Locomotion and Body Form

A STUDY OF GRAVITY AND MAN

BY
DUDLEY J. MORTON, M.D.
Formerly Associate Professor, Department of Anatomy; also Associate Clinical Professor, College of Physicians and Surgeons, Columbia University

With the collaboration of
DUDLEY DEAN FULLER
Associate Professor, Department of Mechanical Engineering, Columbia University

THE WILLIAMS & WILKINS COMPANY
BALTIMORE · 1952

Title page of Dr. Morton's 1952 book Human Locomotion and Body Form.

say that external events like prolonged periods of standing or abusive use due to high heels, do not affect the foot in our youth.[3]

How a Morton's Toe Makes You Hurt

In the following chapters, I will explain specific painful conditions of the foot and body caused by Morton's Toe. But for now, let me tell you how a short first metatarsal bone or hypermobility of the metatarsal bone can cause these problems.

The Short First Metatarsal Bone

In Chapter 22 of his book (see Appendix page 195), *The Human Foot,* Dr. Morton stated that the first metatarsal bone must be at least as long as the second metatarsal

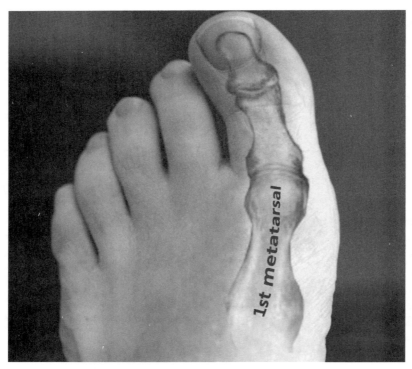

Outline on top of foot showing where first metatarsal bone is.

bone in order for the foot to work properly. When the first metatarsal bone is shorter, it can't do its job of absorbing the stress on the forefoot from walking, standing, and when pushing away from the ground.[4]

What Goes Wrong

In a perfect situation, Mother Nature makes the first metatarsal bone as long as or longer than the second metatarsal bone. "Mom" also designed the first metatarsal bone so that it would be able to carry twice the weight as the second metatarsal bone. However if the first metatarsal bone is shorter than the second metatarsal bone, then this proper lifting by the first metatarsal bone cannot take place.[5] This is because with every step, the second metatarsal bone will abnormally meet the ground before the first metatarsal bone does. When this happens, the first metatarsal bone is blocked from doing its job of supporting most of the weight of the front part of the foot. The second metatarsal bone is now forced to not only lift its share of the burden, but now is made to absorb the first metatarsal bone's share, as well. This makes the second metatarsal bone do 100% of the work, when normally it would be doing only 33% of the work. This puts a tremendous amount of abnormal stress on the second metatarsal bone. It is this "super stress" put upon the second metatarsal bone that starts the chain of events that can cause us to hurt all over.[6]

In other words, in order for our feet to work properly, both metatarsal bones must be on the "same sheet of music," so to speak, every time you take a step. They must work together side by side, holding hands—I mean feet—into the sunset.

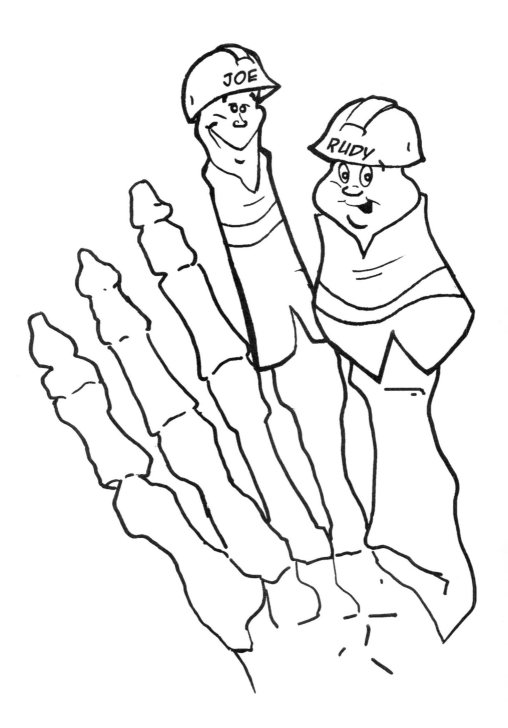

Joe and Rudy

Imagine you are "Joe," the second metatarsal bone. You were hired on for the job of "supporting the foot" and were promised that you would have a full-time co-worker named "Rudy." Rudy is the first metatarsal bone, and he was supposed to be doing twice the heavy lifting on the job, as you, Joe, were. But, Rudy never shows up for work on time and is always a split second late when you need his help supporting the front part of the foot. This doesn't make you, Joe, the second metatarsal bone, a happy camper! Because Rudy is a "no show," you, Joe, are now forced to do 100% of the work of supporting the foot when your job was only supposed to be only 33% of that work. This abnormal strain placed upon you because "Rudy" doesn't show up for work on time forces you, Joe, the second metatarsal bone into a early retirement.

Self-Testing for a Short First Metatsal Bone

One of the ways that the short first metatarsal bone causes damage is by affecting a joint located deep down in the middle of your foot. This joint is where the base of the second metatarsal bone meets the middle cuneiform bone. The base of the second metatarsal bone is located at the opposite end of the bone from where it attaches to the toe bone. On a day-in, day-out basis, people rarely, if ever, complain of any pains in this area.

The drawing on page 28 is from *The Human Foot*, where Morton wanted to show his readers exactly where this painful area was (Fig. 3-1). Part of my normal examination of the foot is to apply pressure directly to this spot, in order to see if there is any tenderness. Because this joint is buried deep down in the foot, patients would normally never be aware if they had a problem with it. Under ordinary circumstances, this area would not hurt. But, if this area is irritated due to a constant Morton's Toe, the patient could have a great deal of pain there. This pain is caused by a synovitis★, or an inflammation/swelling of the joint lining caused by years of abnormal stress and strain going through it.

You can check for yourself if you have this problem. Mentally draw a straight line down from your second toe to the middle of your arch. Look at the picture to the right. It gives you a pretty good idea of where to start. Starting at that point, begin fanning out to exam an area about the size of a half dollar.

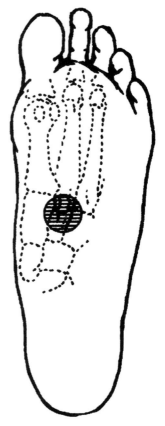

Fig. 3-1. Location of tender joint due to Morton's Toe at the 2nd metatarsal. (Courtesy Columbia University Press.)

Push down with your thumb firmly because the joint we are looking for is deep down in your foot. Make sure your thumb is flat and your finger nail is not digging into the skin (Fig. 3-2.)

You normally should not feel anything more than pressure, but if you do feel some pain or discomfort, there is a good chance that you have some changes in this joint This means that your second metatarsal bone has been

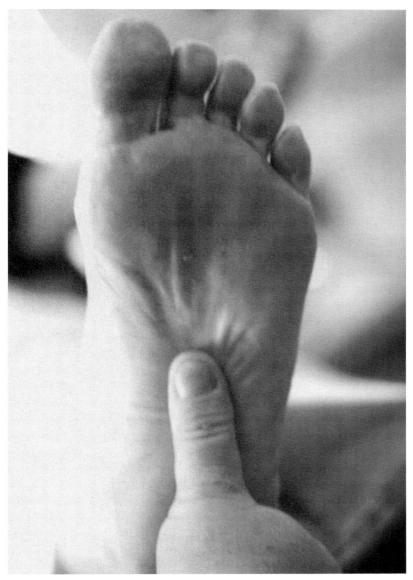

Fig. 3-2. Notice how thumb is flat (not finger nail) as it pushes down to check for pain at the base of the second metatarsal bone.

under a large amount of abnormal stress for some time; most probably due to a short first metatarsal bone.

Remember, in a Morton's Toe because of a short first metatarsal bone, abnormal stress is transferred to the second metatarsal bone; that is why the joint hurts.[7] If you don't have the tenderness at that spot, don't assume you don't have a problem with your feet. It just may mean it hasn't gotten bad enough yet to hurt at that joint.

Hypermobility of the First Metatarsal Bone

In a 1928 paper in the *Journal of Bone and Joint Surgery,* and in Chapter 23 of *The Human Foot* (see Appendix at page 207), Dr. Morton writes about the other problems associated with Morton's Toe.

Hypermobility of the First Metatarsal Bone, may not be as famous as its "partner in pain," the short first metatarsal bone, but in Morton's own words "is responsible for the widest range of foot problems."[8]

Hypermobility refers to the excessive motion present at the first metatarsal bone.

In the normal foot, there would be very little motion at this area. But in a foot with hypermobility of the first metatarsal bone, there is an excessive amount of motion that takes place. According to Dr. Morton, the reason for the excessive motion is due to an abnormal laxity (looseness) of the plantar ligament★ that runs under the metatarsal bone. This laxity is either inherited or acquired in childhood. Because the ligament is abnormally loose, the first metatarsal bone is not as stable as it should be, resulting in many foot problems.[9]

How Important is This?

Hypermobility of the first metatarsal bone is the real cause of the granddaddy of all foot problems, "fallen arches" (Fig. 3-3). As Dr. Morton wrote in *The Human Foot*,

> "Laxity of the plantar ligaments of this seg-
> ment affects both the longitudinal arch, by
> impairing the stability of the foot as a base
> of support, and the fore part of the foot, by
> causing an improper distribution of weight
> upon the metatarsal bones.[10]

In other words if you do have hypermobility at the first metatarsal bone, you will have improper weight bearing, and in turn, will lose the stability needed in supporting

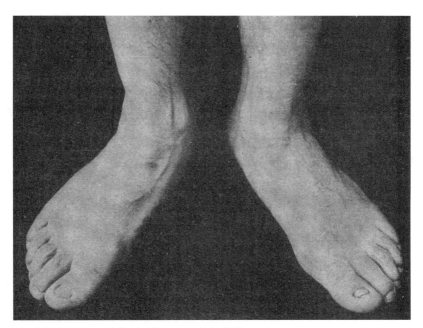

Fig. 3-3. This is what "real fallen arches" look like.

the arch. This is the real reason why our arches fall and is the cause of flat feet.

How many times in your life have you heard the term "fallen arches" and had no idea what it really meant? Now, the next time you are sitting around with friends or family and someone mentions fallen arches, you can impress the heck out of him by saying, "Did you know that according to Professor Dudley Joy Morton, fallen arches are caused by the laxity of the plantar ligaments, causing a hypermobility of the first metatarsal bone, which affects the stability of the longitudinal arch?"

Besides fallen arches, hypermobility of the first metatarsal bone is also responsible for other conditions of the foot and body that will be discussed in Chapters 5, 6, and 7.

Shortness and/or hypermobility of the first metatarsal bone is a two-headed monster that decreases the ability of the first metatarsal to work properly. It causes over-pronation when walking and results in putting greater stress and strain not only on the foot but also on the whole body. In the next chapter, I will explain what over pronation is and how it takes place and adversely affects us.

The Chain Reaction

Just like that old song "Dry Bones," that I presented on page xxi in front of the book, "the foot bone is connected to the head bone." The feet are the foundation of our body in the same way the floor is a foundation of a house. If the floor of your house is not level, the walls won't be straight, the roof will be tilted, and the windows and doors won't close right. The same thing happens with our body. If the foundation of our body is not right because of a Morton's Toe it will tend to make the whole body to get out of alignment. That is why having a problem at the first metatarsal bone can make your back, knees, hip, legs, and even your teeth hurt (Chapter 12). In the following chapters, I will explain this in greater detail.

Chapter 4

Pronation, Morton's Toe and How the Foot Works

Before I tell you about all of the aches and pains that Morton's Toe can cause, I need to tell you about pronation.

> "Pronation has long been recognized as a cardinal sign of foot disorder."
>
> Dr. Dudley J. Morton
> Human Locomotion & Body Form[1]

Pronation is the single most important term used in any discussion of how the foot works. Morton's Toe will cause you to have abnormal or over pronation. This is the cause of most of the problems that I write about, not only of your foot but of your whole body.

What is Pronation?

Pronation is a series of movements our foot must make in order for us to walk properly. But it is not that simple.

There are two types of Pronation of the foot:
1) normal Pronation, or
2) abnormal, or over Pronation

Normal Pronation is a series of motions the foot must

have so that it can absorb the shock of meeting the ground. It must be able to do this in order to adapt and adjust to the new walking surfaces it has just met. This adjustment should only last a fraction of a second to allow the foot to slow down, absorb the shock of your body weight, and adapt to the walking surface. At the point in time when normal pronation is taking place, the foot is referred to as a "Bag of Bones" due to its ability to adapt to the new walking or running surfaces. Part of this process of becoming a "Bag of Bones" is that the arch will start to flatten out and roll toward the ground. Once this adaptation process has taken place, your foot should stop pronating. If this does not happen and your foot keeps "over" pronating, it can then be the start of all the bad things that can happen to your foot and your body. If you think you have "fallen arches" it is most probably because your feet are over pronating.

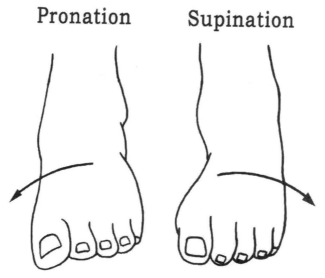

Fig. 4-1. Pronation: In order to become a "Bag of Bones" to adapt to the ground, the arch of the foot rolls down to the ground. Supination: In order to become a rigid lever so it can push off from the ground, the arch rolls up away from the ground.

Over or Abnormal Pronation: As I stated above, this occurs when the foot is still pronating when it shouldn't be. Once the foot has adapted to the ground, the foot should stop pronating and should be starting to stabilizing itself or locking itself. This locking is called Supination* and is the opposite of Pronation. Supination must take place so the foot can become a "Rigid Lever*" (opposite of "Bag of Bones") in order for it to support our body when we push off and away from the ground; and propel us forward for our next step. In Supination, the arch of the foot goes up (instead of down as in Pronation) so that it can become the Rigid Lever. But, if you are "Over-Pronating" and you still are a "Bag of Bones" and not the "Rigid Lever" when pushing off from the ground, then your foot and body will attempt to stop the over prona-tion by compensation.* (Fig. 4-1.)

This compensation* puts the bones, muscles, tendons, ligaments, and other structures under a tremendous amount of abnormal stress and strain not only of the foot but of the whole body. It is this abnormal stress caused by the body attempting to compensate that is the start of most of our feet and body wide problems.

Super Quick Review

This is important, so allow me to repeat the above:

1. When your foot/heel first hits the ground it must be able to pronate in order to be a "bag of bones" so that the foot can adapt to the walking surface.

2. Then, right after it adapts to the ground, the foot must stop pronating, and must start supinating, so that

it can become a "rigid lever" in order to support your foot and whole body when you are pushing off from the ground.

3. But, if at that moment, your foot is not becoming the required rigid lever and still is pronating, then your foot will attempt to fix to this problem by excessive compensation.

4. It is this compensation which makes the body work abnormally that causes our woes, not only of the foot but all over your body.

How the Morton's Toe Causes Compensation

We know that a short first metatarsal bone will cause a lack of proper stabilization on the forefoot, at the critical moment when the foot must be a rigid lever in order for it to push off from the ground. This instability will force the foot to compensate in its attempt to become that rigid lever.

Hypermobility of the first metatarsal bone will cause the same problems as the short first metatarsal bone. By definition, hypermobility of the first metatarsal bone means there is an instability on the front part of the foot, causing improper weight bearing to take place. Because of this instability, the foot has no choice but to compensate in order to become the rigid lever. It is these abnormal forces that start the chain of events, through compensation, that ends in your numerous aches and pains not only of your foot but also throughout your body (Fig. 4-2). Pronation can also be made worse if you have one leg shorter than the other.

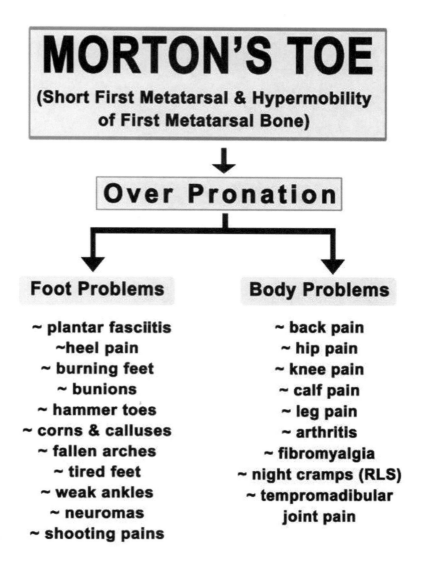

Fig 4-2. This diagram shows how a Morton's Toe can cause over pronation, which then causes pain of the feet and all over the body.

Heel Problems and Pronation

It is universally accepted that over or abnormal Pronation is the most common reason for most heel problems. Pronation causes an excessive pulling, straining, and stretching of the plantar fascia and other structures. It is through these irregular movements of the foot that we can get plantar fasciitis, heel spurs and most of our other heel conditions. In Chapter 6, I will write more about the heel and pronation.

Chapter 5

Conditions of the Foot Caused by Morton's Toe

Since you now know about the two conditions that are associated with Morton's Toe, let's see what foot problems they can cause. Because there are many heel problems, I have devoted the entire next chapter to them. In this chapter, I will deal with the other common foot problems associated with Morton's Toe. I will show you how to treat these problems yourself by using the Toe Pad or Shoe Insert in Chapter 8.

Problems of the Forefoot or Ball of the Foot

The most common foot problems caused by Morton's Toe occur on the ball of the foot. This is because if the first metatarsal bone is short, or is hypermobile, it puts abnormal stress on the ball of the foot. When this happens, the second through fifth metatarsal bones push down abnormally against the ground. Because of this, skin, nerves, muscles, and bursas★ at the ball of the foot can be injured. This can cause the ball to burn, ache, hurt and throb. You can have these pains with or without a callus being present. But the most common problem is a callus under the second metatarsal bone.

Many people, including doctors, believe that burning and pain on the balls of the feet are mostly caused by wearing the wrong shoes. No way! The one thing I do know for sure is that the vast majority of burning or pain on the ball of the foot is caused by Morton's Toe not due to shoes. My strong belief in this matter comes from the thousands of patients and their foot X-rays I have examined over the years. The patients who have come to see me with burning and/or pain on the balls of their feet "almost always" had a short or hypermobile first metatarsal bone on X-ray. When I say almost always, I mean at least 90% of the time. The other 10% of the burning came from diabetes, back problems, or other foot conditions.

It is very common for the burning discomforts or aches to start on the balls of the feet and then spread into the toes or up the legs. Many patients have these leg problems, and it disturbs their sleep. Dr. Morton said these "spasms" at night would occur if great enough strain was put upon the leg muscles caused by hypermobility of the first metatarsal bone[1].

The single most dramatic and impressive result I see from using the Toe Pad is in treating the burning, aches, and pains on the ball of the foot. Most patients tell me there is almost an instant improvement on the ball after we apply the Toe Pad. This is because the simple little Toe Pad realigns the whole front part of the foot and allows it to work properly.

Do You Really Have Nerve Damage Due to Diabetes or Just Bad Feet?

Please allow me to tell you this story. Suppose you are a diabetic, and like millions of other diabetics, you are most likely either on a special diet and/or taking some oral medication or insulin. One day, you go see your doctor for a scheduled appointment. He could be a general practitioner, an internist or an endocrinologist (diabetes specialist); it does not matter. In passing, you mention that you have some burning or pain on the balls of your feet. Your doctor is concerned about this because burning, pain or numbness of the feet is a frequent complication of diabetes. He may think that you are now having serious nerve changes caused by the diabetes, which are called Diabetic Neuropathies. Based on his training and experience, this is a perfectly normal assumption by your doctor.

At that point, your doctor will most likely do one of two things. He might send you to a neurologist (nerve specialist) to be examined, or he might write you a prescription. After several months of taking the medication, one of two things occurs. You either feel better, or you continue to have burning or other discomforts on the balls of your feet. If you still have burning, you go back to your doctor, and he will most probably tell you to increase the dose of your medicine.

But, there is another possible reason for your feet to burn or hurt if you are a diabetic. I have been a professional member of the American Diabetes Association for the majority of the years I have been a foot specialist. Because of that, I do have a pretty good understanding of diabetic neuropathies. What I have seen and believe is that the burning pain, especially on the balls of the feet of fairly healthy and well-managed diabetics, very often is due to Morton's Toe and not due to diabetic neuropathies.

Of course, there are those people who will develop nerve damage from their diabetes, but typically, these patients have been diabetics for many years, and have not taken care of themselves. This is not the average diabetic.

What I am trying to say is that if you are a diabetic, and your feet burn or hurt, it is very possible that it is not caused by nerve damage from your sugar levels, but rather, it is due to the fact that you have a pair of crummy feet—you picked the wrong parents!

It is very possible that many diabetics are taking medications that are not benefiting them when what they really need is to treat their burning, painful feet is a simple Toe Pad. Many physicians are simply not aware of what I just told you. In fact, they would be happy and eager to know that there was another treatment, other than medication, for their diabetic patients with burning feet. Regardless, you need to find out. If you are a diabetic, of any type, you should see your podiatrist at least once a year. He will then be able to evaluate your feet. Then you will know if your problems are due to bad feet or to diabetic nerve complications, or both.

Calluses – What are They and Why Do You Get Them?

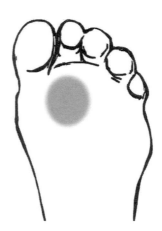

Callus on the ball of the foot

Fig. 5-1. Callus on bottom of 2nd metatarsal head most often caused by Morton's Toe.

A Morton's Toe, in its attempt to make the foot work properly, can cause the second through fifth metatarsal bones to abnormally push down against the ground. To protect us against this abnormal pushing down, Mother Nature makes a protective thickening of the skin (shock absorber), when needed under the affected metatarsal heads. This thickening of the skin is called a *callus* (Fig. 5-1). The most common location for calluses is under the second metatarsal head. But they can also appear under the third, fourth or fifth metatarsal heads. Over a period of time, and with enough abnormal pressure, the skin under the callus can break down and cause an ulcer★. Like most foot problems, calluses can be made worse by poor shoes. However unless you have a short first metatarsal bone or a hypermobility of the first metatarsal bone to start with, you won't have calluses as readily.

Corns

A corn is a hard abnormal thickening of the skin that develops on the top, sides or in between the toe bones, because of repeated friction and pressure. Like a callus, a

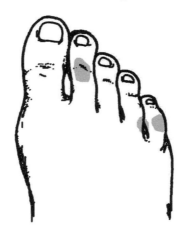

Corns & Soft Corns

Fig. 5-2. Corns are caused by hammer toes, and most often occur on the top or side of the 5th toes. The 2nd toes are also a common place for corns. Soft corns most commonly occur between the 4th and 5th toes and at the toe web.

corn is another one of Mother Nature's shock absorbers. They can appear at numerous places on the toes, but, the top and side of the fifth toe is the most common. A soft corn is caused by pressure or friction in between the toes or in the toe webs in combination with perspiration. Because moisture is always present, this corn tissue does not have an opportunity to harden and stays soft (Fig. 5-2).

What Causes Corns?

Corns can be caused by wearing shoes that do not fit right. But I feel they can also be caused by having a Morton's Toe. This is what happens. We know that as a result of Morton's Toe, the metatarsal bones will push down on the ground in an attempt to bear weight properly. This is how calluses are formed. When the metatarsal bones are pushing down, the tendons on the top of the toes of these metatarsal bones will pull up and abnormally tighten. The tendons on the bottom of the toes will also work abnormally. This causes the toe to "hammer," or go up in the shoe. When this happens, the toes will start to rub against the top of the shoe. It is this hammering, inside of the shoe, that with time, can cause the recurrent friction and pressure that leads to corns. The action where the metatarsal bone goes down, and the toes go up, is like a seesaw and is called "retrograde force."

Put your three middle fingers under the ball of either foot. Now, with your other hand, pull your toes all the way down. When you do this, you should feel that the metatarsal heads move up, away from the bottom of your feet. Do this several more times until you see that the metatarsal bones are going up into your feet when you pull your toes down.

Now, the important part: do the exact opposite. Put your fingers back on the ball of your foot, but now pull your toes up. It should be very easy for you to feel that the heads of the metatarsal bones are now pushing down. The metatarsal bones are bulging out, toward the ball of your foot. They are very prominent and should be easy to find. The metatarsal heads can feel like bumps, rocks or stones on the bottom of the feet. This is important, so please allow me to repeat it again.

When your metatarsal bones are pushed down against the ground abnormally because of Morton's Toe, they are not only the cause of calluses. This force is causing the tendons on the top of the toes to tighten, causing a "hammer toe." When these abnormal hammer toes are put into even a good shoe, it can cause recurrent friction and pressure to occur on the toes. That is how corns can and do form. As I said before, by using a Toe Pad, you can keep the hammer toe from forming in the first place.

What are Bunions?

A simple or moderate bunion is an abnormal bump of bone that is formed at the head of our old friend, the first metatarsal bone (Fig. 5-3). The bunion can either be on the top or side of the first metatarsal bone. In a more advanced bunion deformity, called *Hallux Abducto Valgus*★, there starts to be a movement of the big toe toward the second toe (Fig. 5-4). The most severe bunion is when the first toe not only moves toward the second toe, but starts to overlaps or under laps the second toe.

If a simple bunion bump is formed, there is a good chance Mother Nature will step in and produce a shock absorber that will protect the bunion bump. This shock absorber is called a bursa. A bursa is a fluid-containing sac. With time and enough irritation, the sac (bursa) that is protecting the bunion can become swollen, inflamed, and sore. This problem is known as *bursitis*★.

Why We Get Bunions

Over the years, the one constant that I have seen with patients who have bunions is a short first metatarsal bone and/or hypermobility of the first metatarsal bone, due to inheritance. We know that Morton's Toe takes place at the first metatarsal bone, so it makes sense you will have a lot of abnormal stresses and strains at that area. Because of this, bunions can and do exist.

A lot has been written about how shoes are a major cause of bunions. I can agree with that only up to a point. Believe it or not, at one time or another there are some people who insist on wearing shoes that are incorrect for

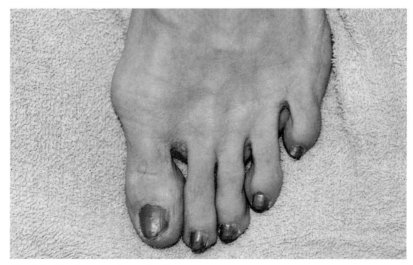

Fig. 5-3. Simple or moderate bunion.

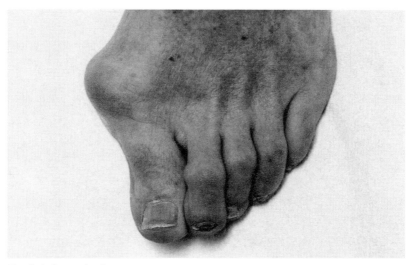

Fig. 5-4. Severe bunion.

them. Do all of these people have bunions or other foot problems? Of course not. The ones who end up getting foot problems are the ones born with the poor combination of having a short metatarsal bone, and/or hypermobility of the first metatarsal bone. The truth is, though, if you insist on constantly wearing shoes that are not right for you, then there is a strong likelihood that you not only will get bunions, but most of the other problems in this book, regardless of how normal your feet are. In any case, if your bunions don't hurt, leave them alone.

Fallen Arches, Weak Ankles, Ankle Sprains and Tired Feet

Everybody knows or has heard of "fallen arches". The million dollar question is: why do we get fallen arches to start with?

The Why

Dr. Morton wrote passionately about the true causes of fallen arches, tired feet, and weak ankles in his article of 1928[2], and his books of 1935[3], 1939[4] and 1952.[5] He had no doubt that all of these problems were caused by the hypermobility of the first metatarsal bone. He said there was a loss of stability at the arch when you had hypermobility of the first metatarsal bone. This loss of stability will then cause the arch to fall, tilt or collapse inwardly because it has less support than normal in keeping the arch up.

Once this collapsing starts toward the inside part of the foot, then a chain reaction begins to take place that can cause many problems of your foot, heel and ankle. The muscles of the ankle will attempt to fight off this unnatural inward titling or collapsing of the arch. But if the abnormal forces put upon the muscles at the ankle and at the arch are too great, then these muscles will become strained and exhausted. They will then start to hurt in their attempt to prevent the arch from collapsing and to maintain the balance of the feet.[6]

This unsuccessful battle of trying to prevent the arch from collapsing by the muscles of the ankle is also a common cause of tired feet and weak ankles. Chronic ankle sprains can also be caused by this acquired instability at the ankle joint due to its battle of trying to prevent the arch from collapsing.[7] This straining or exhausting of the muscles can also cause spasms at night.[8] The good news is that these problems can be easily treated with a Toe Pad or a Shoe Insert. In reality, true "fallen arches" are a rare thing. In spite of the fact that the term is now used to refer to several foot problems, in actuality it means a total break-down and substantial deformity of the foot. This severe condition is, in fact, a truly uncommon occurrence in our time.

The Neuroma of Dr. Thomas G. Morton – What is a Neuroma?

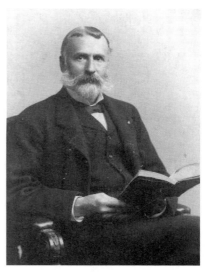

In 1876, Dr. Thomas G. Morton, of the Pennsylvania Hospital, presented a new medical condition that was called a *neuroma.*[9] A neuroma is an abnormal thickening or swelling of a nerve, resulting in shooting pains into the toes or ball of the foot. The nerve we are most

Dr. Thomas G. Morton, about 1890 (Courtesy University of Pennsylvania Health System.)

concerned about in a neuroma is the medial *plantar nerve,* which lies between the 3rd and 4th metatarsal bones (Fig. 5-5). It is highly unlikely that Dr. Dudley J. Morton ever met Dr. Thomas Morton because Thomas died in 1903, when Dudley was just starting medical school. They were not related. However Morton's Toe, and Morton's Neuroma do have a great deal in common, as you will see a couple of pages down the road.

How a Morton's Toe Causes a Morton's Neuroma

Morton's Neuroma is caused by an abnormal irritation of the nerve that takes place over a period of time. This irritation to the nerve is caused by excessive pressure, motion or trauma to the front part of the foot. But what causes this excessive pressure, motion or trauma to begin with? Can it have something to do with Morton's Toe? You bet! As I wrote previously, in *The Agony Of De-Feet:*

> This painful foot condition (neuroma) is due to a choking off of the nerves that run through the foot. The nerves are choked by the metatarsal bones, which are being improperly squeezed together due to an abnormal motion in the foot, generally (due to) hereditary.[10]

I did not realize that over 25 years ago, I was giving my (then) readers the exact description of how a Morton's Toe could cause a Morton's neuroma. The improper squeezing of the medial plantar nerve by the metatarsal bones as described above can be caused by any of the lesser metatarsal bones, but most often is caused by the 3rd and 4th bones.

In his 1927 article[11] and his 1935 book,[12] Dudley Morton explained how Morton's Neuroma can occur due to failures of the first metatarsal bone. Morton also wrote that one of the areas of the foot that receives the greatest amount of abnormal stress and strain due to Morton's Toe is located at the joint formed by the second metatarsal bone with the second cuneiform bone (Fig. 3-1). Because of the constant pulling, tearing and tugging of these two bones, the joint is literally pulling itself apart. Morton believed that since the nerve involved in Morton's Neuroma is located in close proximity to this joint, it (the nerve) can also get irritated by the joint's improper motion. This motion can cause some of the pain associated with Morton's Neuroma.

You Really Need to Sit Down for This

If further proof is still needed that a Morton's Toe can cause a Morton's Neuroma, we need to go no further

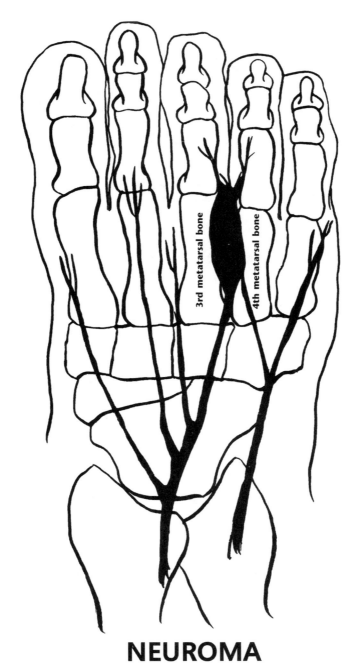

3rd metatarsal bone

4th metatarsal bone

NEUROMA

Fig. 5-5. A neuroma is a swollen nerve most commonly caused by the 3rd and 4th metatarsal bone (heads) choking the nerve.

than to consult Dr. Thomas George Morton, "Father of the Neuroma." Okay, bear with me here because it does get slightly confusing. Remember, Dr. Thomas Morton first wrote about the neuroma of the foot in 1876.[13] Some fifty years later, in 1927, Dr. Dudley Morton wrote about the problems caused by the short first metatarsal bone, including neuroma, for the very first time in the *Journal of Bone and Joint Surgery*.[14] Dr. Thomas G. Morton died in 1903. That was about twenty-five years before the first paper on Morton's Toe was ever published by Dr. Dudley Morton. So, how could Dr. Thomas G. Morton, who was very dead in 1927 and had been for almost twenty-five years, confirm that Morton's Toe was a cause of his neuroma? Are you still with me? I warned you to sit down.

This is how. In 1896, Dr. Thomas G. Morton wrote a paper for the *International Medical Magazine*. In it, he presented two case histories in regard to his metatarsalgia, or neuroma. With the case histories, he included foot X-rays to help explain and support what he was writing about in his article.[15] Guess what one of those X-rays showed? It showed a short first metatarsal bone! Not any short first metatarsal bone but one of the shortest first metatarsal bones I have ever seen![16] (Fig. 5-6.)

This X-ray was reproduced by Dudley Morton in his 1927 paper[17] and again in *The Human Foot* in 1935.[18] It was presented to show how the Morton's Toe can be the cause of Morton's Neuroma. It is not everyday that one doctor who was dead for a quarter of a century can confirm the work of another doctor! But that's what Thomas Morton M.D. did for Dudley Morton M.D. when he included those X-rays of that very short first metatarsal bone in his 1896 paper.

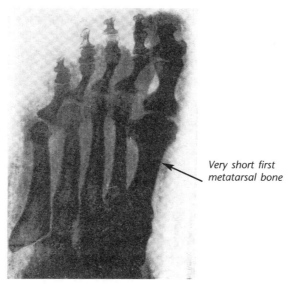

Very short first
metatarsal bone

Fig. 5-6. Dr. Thomas G. Morton 1896 X-ray showing the short first metatarsal bone as the cause of the "Morton's Neuroma" (Int. Medical Magazine).

Self Test for Morton's Neuroma

It is fairly simple to see if you do have a Morton's Neuroma. Look at Fig. 5-7.

The area circled is called the base of the 3rd interspace of the foot. This is the spot where the swelling of the nerve (neuroma) most often occurs in the foot.

Now press down at that marked area on the top of your foot with your second finger.

Using your thumb, press on the bottom of your foot directly under the spot where you are pressing on the top of your foot. You may need to move the fingers around a little on the top and bottom of the foot and you will need to squeeze hard. But if you have a neuroma, you will know it from the discomfort you feel. If you do feel pain, I will show you how to treat it yourself by making the Toe Pad in Chapter 8.

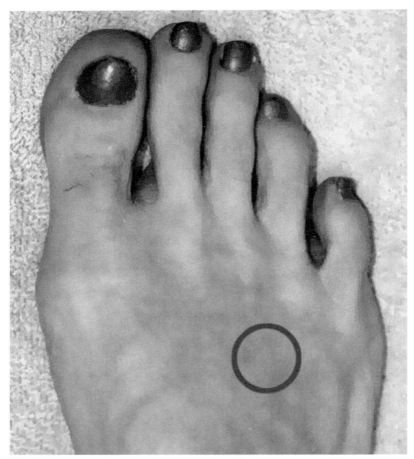

Fig. 5-7. Circled area is common location for neuroma between the 3rd and 4th metatarsal bones.

Arthritis

Almost every day a patient will ask me, "Doc, do I have arthritis in my feet?" My answer is, "If you can remember watching the *Ed Sullivan Show* on television, then you most probably have some form of arthritis in your feet or somewhere else in your body." Most of the foot problems written about in this book are one form of arthritis or another.

What is Arthritis?

According to the Arthritis Foundation, there are over one hundred types of arthritis.[19] It is a disease that affects the joints and the soft tissues in and around the joints. A joint is the place where two bones meet. The most common form of bony arthritis that affects the body and the foot is called osteoarthritis.★ This occurs when the joint is broken down from "wear and tear" over a period of years. There are other types of arthritis that do not attack the joints, however. These types of arthritis are called "non-articulating arthritis" and are inflammatory conditions. They affect the soft tissue as opposed to the bones. These soft tissue (non bone) arthritis types are the most common foot problems that I see on a daily basis. They include such problems as bursitis★, fasciitis★, capsulitis★, and synovitis★.

What Causes Arthritis in the Feet?

Many things can cause arthritis in the feet but either directly or indirectly, it is caused a great deal of the time by Morton's Toe. If your foot is constantly being abused on a day-in day-out basis due to a Morton's Toe or other foot problems, sooner or later the damage to these joints and other soft tissue structures will end up giving you some form of arthritis.

The $0.75 Pad or the $7,500.00 Surgery?

A common place for arthritis to appear in the foot because of Morton's Toe is at the big toe joint. This joint is called the first metatarsal phalange joint. It is where the first metatarsal bone connects with the big toe. This arthritis can cause decreased motion at the big toe joint, resulting in a great deal of pain and swelling. The medical term for this condition is *Hallux Limitus*. During my career, I have seen many different surgeries to repair the damage done by arthritis to the big toe joint.

Like most doctors, I am called upon by representatives of drug companies or medical equipment companies. Not too long ago, a nice gentleman from one of these equipment companies came to see me. He was there to tell me about a new surgical device and surgery to repair the damage done to the big toe joint due to arthritis of the joint. He played a DVD that showed the surgery and his new device. The surgery removed the old destroyed cartilage* at the head of the first metatarsal bone and replaced it with a state-of-the-art titanium-coated implant in its place. It was great! It was wonderful! I really think this implant and surgery are going to work and help a lot of people. I told the representative what I thought, and he seemed very pleased. He then invited me to a hands-on workshop to learn how to perform the surgery. I thanked him for the invitation but told him my philosophy of practice was geared toward preventing problems so surgeries were not necessary. I told him that if the patient in his DVD had placed a simple little pad under his first metatarsal bone as recently as three to five years ago, the arthritis that destroyed his big toe joint probably would not have happened, or at worst, would have been more manageable. He gave me a blank look and said, "I didn't know that." I said, "Yeah, I know; I get that a lot." Again, I told him I thought he had a winner with this new device, but only time would tell for sure. I also suggested that he recommend to all of the doctors that he would would later visit after the implant surgery, that they also treat the underlying real problem of the Morton's Toe. If they didn't do that, the surgery could fail.

The point of this story is this. It is marvelous we have these new surgeries and devices to repair these conditions. However, if the patient in the DVD or his doctor knew about the work of Dr. Dudley Morton, that patient might not have ever been in the DVD to start with. Moreover, he could have saved thousands of dollars, not to mention the discomfort and inconvenience caused by the surgery.

March or Stress Fractures

Another problem that I believe is caused by a Morton's Toe is a spontaneous breaking (fracture) of the lesser metatarsal bone(s), most commonly the second metatarsal bone. In the military, these fractures called "march fractures." In the private world they are called stress fractures (Fig. 5-9). When military recruits go on marches, some of them end up with fractures of their second metatarsal bone for no apparent reason. I would bet anything that if the X-rays were re-examined on these men, they would show that the majority of the ones who got a march fracture also had a short or hypermobile first metatarsal bone. Again, it makes sense. If you have either of these problems, the poor lesser metatarsal bone, especially the second, has a lot more stress and strain on it than the normal foot would have. Add to that a 60-pound backpack and double-time march, and it's no wonder the unfortunate second metatarsal bone breaks. I believe it would be of great benefit to our armed forces for their doctors to consider this relationship between the first metatarsal bone and march fractures. If they did, two things would occur:

1. The number of march fractures would drop markedly, and

2. Thousands and thousands of cases of various foot, back, leg, neck, and hip problems associated with the Morton's Toe would also decrease, saving our country millions of dollars in treating our armed forces.

In the civilian world, a stress fracture is the same thing as the march fracture except it is caused by day-in day-out stress applied upon the metatarsal bone and not by marching. I have found that dancing, jogging and golfing many times will cause it. In both the march fracture and the stress fracture it is very common that there are no signs on X-rays of the break of the metatarsal bone for several weeks. So it is common that the foot must be re-X-rayed to observe the fracture. In my office, I am fortunate because I have the use of diagnostic ultrasound (the same

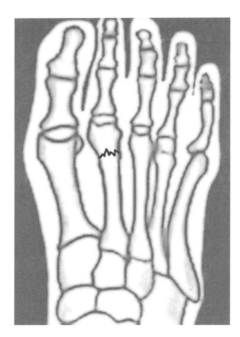

Fig. 5-9 The broken line at the 2nd metatarsal bone shows a common location of March or Stress Fractures.

type of machine used by obstetricians to watch babies grow). This allows me, to see the fracture immediately without having to wait several weeks.

Night Cramps and Restless Legs Syndrome

I ask all of my new patients if they have any problems sleeping because of any discomfort of their legs. Many of them tell me that in fact they are experiencing nightly leg cramps that disturb their sleep. Some also tell me that they are being treated for restless legs syndrome. Night leg cramps are abnormal contractions of the leg muscles. They normally can awaken the patient from a deep sleep. The exact cause of night cramps is not known; however, everything from poor circulation, dehydration, muscle overexertion, imbalance of electrolytes, to drug reactions, has been proposed. Some of the more popular treatments for night cramps have been stretching of the leg muscles, hot packs, cold packs, and massage. For years, quinine was a very popular drug for the treatment of night cramps. But in December 2006, the U.S. Food and Drug Administration took it off the market because of its serious side effects.[20]

Can a Morton's Toe Cause Night Cramps?

Dudley Morton did thought so, and so do I. In *The Human Foot*, he discusses how the hypermobility of the first metatarsal bone can cause spasms and strains in the leg muscles that can then cause disturbances in sleep.[21] If your feet are overworked because of problems at the first metatarsal bone, you can have tired feet, fallen arches, and weak ankles. Because of that, it is not a big leap to see how your leg muscles could also become strained and exhausted and cause night cramps. I regularly treat patients who did have problems sleeping because of night cramps and who told me that their cramps got better when I treated their foot problems. This is different from the patients who also tell me they are just sleeping better because their feet are now hurting less.

Restless Legs Syndrome

According to the National Institutes of Health, Restless Legs Syndrome (RLS) is a neurological disorder characterized by unpleasant sensations in the legs and an uncontrollable urge to move them for relief. Individuals affected with the disorder describe the sensations as burning, creeping, tugging, or like insects crawling inside the legs. The sensations range in severity from uncomfortable to irritating to painful.[22] There is no known cause for this condition, but it does run in families in up to half of the people with RLS. Recently the general public is hearing more about it than ever before. This is because of the TV ads for the new medications for its treatment.

At no time am I saying that Morton's Toe is a cause of RLS. There is no evidence to support this, but, please allow me the opportunity to tell you what is on my mind concerning RLS and Morton's Toe and the possibility there may be some connection between the two. Could it be possible that some of the problems that we see in night cramps, caused by Morton's Toe, such as exhaustion or strain of the leg muscles, are also contributing to the causes of RLS? My answer to this question is "I don't know." What I do know is that the majority of the patients who come to see me with pre-diagnosed (by another physician) RLS do have a short first metatarsal bone and/or hypermobility of the first metatarsal bone. When I treat the problem(s) at the first metatarsal bone, many of these patients tell me their RLS does improve.

Up to now I am not aware of anyone, at any time, questioning the possible relationship between Morton's Toe and Restless Legs Syndrome. But I do believe it is worth asking considering the great benefits that could be gained by determining if there is any correlation between these two problems. According to the RLS Foundation, about nine million people in this country have RLS.[23] Statistically, if only one-tenth of one percent of these people got some relief from RLS by treating their Morton's Toes, 9,000 people could be sleeping better soon.

If you do suffer with either night cramps or RLS, you may want to start using the Toe Pad or Shoe Insert that I describe in Chapter 8. It may take weeks to see a change, but you have nothing to lose and everything to gain. Again, common sense dictates that in any group of people who have night cramps or RLS, some of them are going to have Morton's Toe and all the problems that come with it as well. The problems associated with their Morton's Toes just have to be aggravating the sleeping problems in some of those people. You could be one of them, and you will never know if my suggested treatment for your toes will help you until you try. Regardless, advise your physician that you are trying this because he needs to know if your problems get better or not. Stranger things have happened.

Special Situations

The following situations are not medical conditions like the others in this chapter but are nevertheless important enough to be written about.

High Heel Shoes

During his entire career, Morton repeatedly warned women about the dangers of the excessive wearing of high heel shoes. From the *New York Times*, November 5, 1935:

Women Advised to Limit Wearing of High Heels

If women would wear high heels only during the evening they would suffer far fewer foot disorders according to Dr. Dudley J. Morton, Professor of Anatomy in the Columbia University Medical School. Dr. Morton, in a survey in The Human Foot just published, termed high heel shoes a powerful and vicious factor in the disorder when worn during working hours. He asserted that it was not high heels themselves but continuous use of them that made women more susceptible to foot disorders than men.[24]

Now, it is no great news flash that high heel shoes will make women's feet hurt. What is news, though, is the logical way Morton explains why this pain occurs.

Let's assume you are a woman with a perfectly normal pair of feet. Your first metatarsal bone is nice and long, and all the weight on the ball of your feet is being carried properly by all five of the metatarsal bones. Under normal circumstances, when you walk, your heel is meeting the ground about one-half of the time. This means the ball of your foot is off the ground not bearing any weight the other one-half of the time. However, in high heels, your heel bone is never meeting the ground. The pressure is on the ball of your foot constantly, 100% of the time. Over a period of time, this is bad enough for a woman with normal feet, but if you are a woman who has the classic, short first metatarsal bone, your foot problems have just multiplied in high heels. The reason for this is because not only is the ball of your feet under constant pressure 100% of the time in high heels, but that constant pressure is being carried mostly by the second metatarsal bone. What I am trying to say is that because the weight is never shifted back to the heel at least half of the time, the second metatarsal bone is carrying 100% of the pressure, 100% of the time.[22] This is a recipe for a train wreck waiting to happen in regards to your feet. If you would like to minimize this damage, my recommendation is to wear the Toe Pad directly on the bottom of your first metatarsal bone whenever you wear high heels.

Sports

Like many other well-adjusted men, I am a sports fan. In fact, a day rarely goes by without me tuning in to ESPN★ to see what is going on in football, golf, tennis, basketball or baseball. Be it professional or college, I need my daily fix of sports. What I have noticed is that a week seldom goes by without a report of how one of these outstanding athletes is injured in the foot, ankle or knee. Why would some players get an injury when most don't? They are all wearing the same type of shoes. They all train and play as hard as each other. Like all the other problems I discuss in this book, I absolutely believe that Morton's Toe is the cause of many of these non-contact injuries. I think it would be a great idea if all trainers and team doctors would start to check their players for Morton's Toe. If some players do have a short first metatarsal bone, it would be easy to include Toes Pad in with their feet and ankle strappings that are applied daily. This would make the foot and ankle more stable and cut down on injuries.

Jogging or Running

Beside world class athletes, the average person is much more likely to have sport-related problems because of Morton's Toe. "Boomerist" is a term coined in 1999 by Dr. Nicholas A. DiNubile, an orthopedic surgeon at the University of Pennsylvania, to denote injuries to those who are part of the Baby Boomer generation. As the Baby Boomers get older, they are having more ailments, aches, pains, and injuries than their parents and grandparents because they are much more active. According to the Consumer Product Safety Commission, sports injuries among the baby boom generation increased 33% in the 1990s, contributing to the estimated 17 million sports injuries in America each year.[25]

One of the most popular activities of the Boomers is jogging and/or running. The problem with this activity is that even with normal feet, you will sooner or later tend to have feet, shin, leg, or knee problems. From my experience, if you run over thirty miles a week, there is a good chance that even with good feet (unless you are very lucky), you will have some problems. Hopefully if you are running thirty miles a week or more, you are smart enough to go see your local podiatrist and have a pair of orthotics made for you to PREVENT these problems from occurring. For any serious runner, orthotics is the key to having many years of pain-free running. I have treated world-class runners, tri-athletes and some who run in the Boston Marathon. Prevention is everything.

Now, let's talk about those joggers/runners who don't have a normal foot. If you think you may have some foot problems, don't wait to start using the Toe Pad or Shoe Insert. Use them at once! By doing so, you may delay such problems as Anterior Compartment Syndrome, Overuse Syndrome, Chondromalacia (Runner's Knee) and other problems caused by the constant abuse and pounding on the body brought on by running. If you have already been diagnosed with any of the above, it's time to check out your feet. Baby Boomer or not, our bodies were not designed to take the abuse that can be caused by a Morton's Toe when you are a runner or jogger.

Other Activities

Running is not the only activity that can aggravate a bad foot. Golfing, tennis, ballroom dancing, bowling, softball, and basketball are some of the many pastimes that bring patients into my office. If you are involved any of these activities, or similar activities that may potentially damage your feet, it is important that you see a podiatrist and become proactive regarding your feet. Until then, try the Toe Pad to see if it may help you. As you will see shortly, it is very easy to make and wear, so what have you got to lose? Try it!

Eldridge

On June 18, 2008, Tiger Woods announced that he would not be playing anymore golf in 2008 due to a recurring knee problem. So I must ask the following question: Why would a super healthy guy like Tiger, who is not heavy in any shape or form, have to have four knee surgeries to start with? Tiger has the best surgeons on the planet. So why does this knee problem keep coming back? Is it possible that his knee problem is really starting in his foot? Of course, I don't know. In fact, I might be absolutely, positively, dead wrong. However, I would love to find out if Eldridge's (Tiger's real name) second metatarsal bone was longer than his first metatarsal bone and if his mom or dad have ever had foot problems. It is highly unlikely that any of Tiger's doctors ever considered how a Morton's Toe might be aggravating their patient's knee. What I do know based on the work of Dr. Travell and what I see regularly in my office is that knee problems can be improved greatly by using the Toe Pad. Four knee surgeries is three too many, including one to remove a tumor. So Tiger – try the Toe Pad and let me know how it works for you.

Chapter 6

Heel Problems

The most common foot problems that I see on a daily basis are those that are associated with the heels or arches. The heel is the largest bone in the foot and is designed to handle the most stress, strain, and pressure. It is the workhorse of the foot. Every time we take a step, our entire body weight goes through our heels. Over the course of the day, tons of weight are placed over your heel bone.

Can You Say *Poststatic Dyskinesia?*

I can't, and I have been trying for years. This tongue twister is a very common complaint that patients have when their heels start to hurt them. It is the pain of the heel or the arch that appears when you first get out of bed in the morning. It can also occur upon standing, after resting or sitting for a while, any time during the day. Some patients state that they get this pain upon getting out of their car after driving for a while. *Poststatic Dyskinesia* is most commonly caused by a Plantar Fasciitis or a Heel Bursitis. I can determine how bad a heel condition is by asking the patient how long it takes the pain to go away after getting up. Normally it takes about 5-15 minutes for the heel pain to start to go away. If it takes longer than that, I then know this patient has a very unpleasant heel problem. Another question I ask them is if they have to hold on to something just to get out of bed or to stand up. If they do, I know that I am dealing with a very bad case of heel or arch pain. You can have heel pain any time during the day, but I feel the most common times are in the morning, with pain upon arising from bed or upon standing after resting for a while.

Plantar Fasciitis (Heel Pain Syndrome)

The single most common heel problem seen in this country is *Plantar Fasciitis* or Heel Pain Syndrome. Plantar Fasciitis is an inflammation and/or swelling of the plantar fascia. The plantar fascia is a large, tough, fibrous rubber-band-like structure that holds up the inside part of your foot.

When we talk about the arch of the foot, we are talking about the plantar fascia (Fig. 6-1). It is attached to the bottom side of the heel bone from a projection known as the medial tuberosity. The plantar fascia then travels across the whole bottom of the foot and attaches into the toe bones. The plantar fascia must serve as a platform (rigid level) that braces the foot when walking and allows us to push off away from the ground with our toes. The plantar fascia can be strained for numerous reasons, including Morton's Toe. When this occurs, it can get inflamed, causing Plantar Fasciitis. Like heel bursitis, it can also cause you to have *Poststatic Dyskinesia*.

Heel Bursitis

A bursa is a fluid-containing sac that is present at many areas of pressure on the body. Its job is to protect these areas of pressure by being a shock absorber. A bursitis is

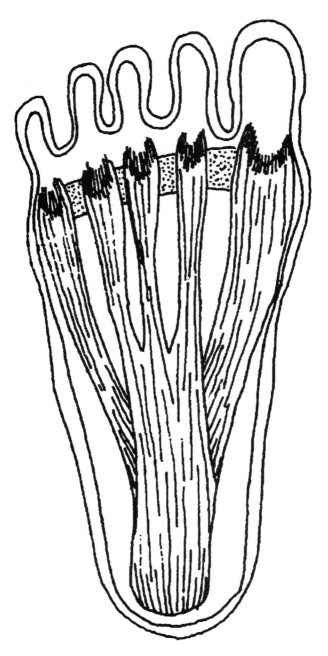

Fig. 6-1. The plantar fascia is the large rubber-band type structure that helps support our whole foot. Because of that, it gets strained a great deal and is the major cause of heel pain.

an abnormal inflammation of the bursa sac caused by abnormal excessive pressure, stress and/or strain over the area it is protecting. On the heel bone, there are two bursa sacs: one on the bottom and the other on the back. Specifically, on the bottom of the heel, it is known as an Inferior (bottom) Calcaneal (heel) Bursa. On the back of the heel, it is called the Retro (back) Calcaneal Bursa.

When either of these bursas become abnormally stressed, strained, or swollen, the result is bursitis of the heel. It is this bursitis that is the reason for pain in the heel upon arising (Poststatic Dyskinesia) in the morning or after resting for a while. You can develop either of these bursitises with or without the presence of heel spurs (explanation to follow). As stated before, Morton's Toe can cause this by causing over pronation in the foot.

Heel Spurs

Heel spurs are abnormal projections of bone growing out from either the bottom or back of the heel. The reason we get heel spurs is the abnormal pulling at the bottom or back of the heel, which is a result of over-pronation, over a period of years. Morton's Toe causes this over-pronation. If this pulling is great enough, it can cause a tearing away of the plantar fascia from where it attaches to the heel. This spot on the bottom of the heel bone is known as the Medial Tuberosity. The tearing away of the plantar fascia from the Medial Tuberosity causes micro-scopic bleeding to occur in this tissue. The tissue that is torn away is called the periosteum.★ When periosteum bleeds, new bone is produced. This new bone is how a heel spur is formed. On the back of the heel, the same thing is happening except it is the Achilles Tendon that is pulled away from the bone and not the Plantar Fascia.

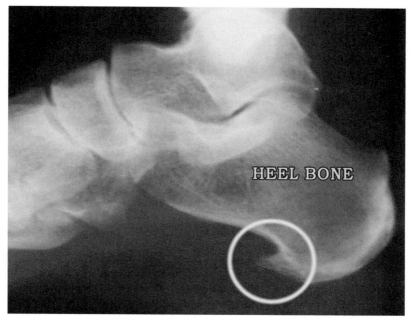

Fig. 6-2. Inside the circle is a large heel spur. Normally they are not this large, but I picked it to show you what they really look like.

On an X-ray, the new spur can appear as a little dot, or with time, as a large fish hook (Fig. 6-2).

Heel Spurs Don't Always Hurt

Right now, as you are reading this book, there are literally millions of people walking the streets, valleys, and dales of this country who have the biggest heel spurs you can imagine (like the one in Fig. 6-2 above). Aside from having these huge heel spurs, these people have one other thing in common. **Their heels do not hurt! That is right. Their heels do not hurt! And guess what? They have no idea that they even have heel spurs!**

It is very common for me to be X-raying a foot for a totally different foot problem and find a heel spur on the

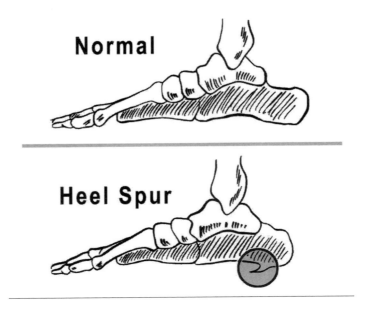

Normal

Heel Spur

X-ray. Upon questioning such patients, they would often tell me that they never suffered one moment with heel pain and were not even aware that they had heel spurs. Furthermore, it is not unusual for me to see a patient who said they had heel pain for about two to three months. On an X-ray, that patient would have a massive spur that from its size would have had to be there for many years. I am of the firm belief that heel spurs can lay dormant for years, until the day comes when you take that one bad step that triggers you to have heel pain. Why then, do many people who have heel spurs go through their entire lives without having any heel pain? It can be pure luck, (remember that one bad step) or it could be due to other factors such as their job, hours standing, weight, or shoes. All these factors can have something to do with crossing that line into having heel pain after an entire life of having none. Regardless of the reason or whether it hurts or not, if you do have a heel spur on X-ray, it tells me that your heel and foot has had to have been under abnormal stress for some time and that they are not working right.

Why the Morton's Toe Can Be the Reason for Plantar Fasciitis, Heel Pain, Heel Spurs, Poststatic Dyskinesia and Lots of Other Stuff

When I first really got interested in the work of Dr. Dudley J. Morton, I was always aggressively investigating to see if his concepts were accurate. Was it really possible that the short first metatarsal bone and/or the hypermobility of the first metatarsal bone could really be responsible for all those foot problems? Since heel troubles were the most common problem I treated, I needed a way to discover if Morton's principles stood up to the test in regard to problems of the heels. Up to that time, and through today, no one that I am aware of has every ever written about the connection between the malfunctions at the first metatarsal bone and heel/arch pain. Despite my best efforts in researching textbooks, journals, articles, and searching the web, I have never found ANYTHING ever written or mentioned about heel pain, heel spurs or plantar fasciitis in relation to Morton's Toe. In fact, if someone has written about this before me, I apologize from the outset for not giving you credit.

Podiatrists will generally take two X-rays views of the heel bone when there are heel or arch complaints. That is how foot specialists are trained, and that is how it is normally done. In order for me to see if Morton's Toe could cause heel pain, I needed to take one additional X-ray view than those that are routinely taken. This X-ray view

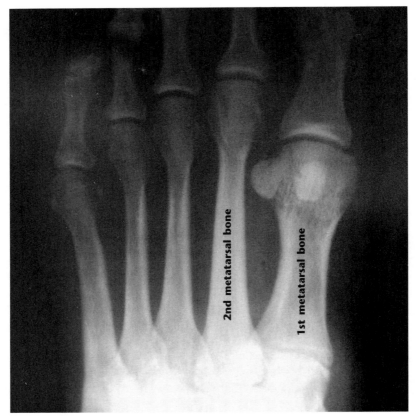

Fig. 6-3. This is called a dorsal plantar view of the foot. It is the most common view used by podiatrists and the one I use to confirm if a patient has a Morton's Toe or not.

is called the *Dorsal Plantar view*, and looks straight down over the foot (Fig. 6-3).

This view allows me to see the length of the patient's first metatarsal bone and determine if there was anything else on the X-ray that was consistent with hypermobility of the first metatarsal bone. In other words, does this patient with heel problems also have a Morton's Toe? Yes, they did! In at least 90% of my patients, X-rays showed that those who had heel spurs, plantar fasciitis, or other heel pains, also had either a short first metatarsal bone and/or other changes consistent with hypermobility of the first metatarsal bone. This finding is much more than a coincidence. Again, I am not aware of anyone making that observation before me.

I invite other professionals to perform similar X–rays on their patients and verify if what I am presenting is true. I believe that they will find a short first metatarsal bone and/or hypermobility of the first metatarsal bone present in the vast majority of their patients with heel or arch pain.

Why?

The reason heel problems arise in the presence of Morton's Toe is fairly straightforward. It all goes back to abnormal pronation that I wrote about in Chapter 4. If you have a Morton's Toe, the front part of the foot is unstable when it needs to be stable. Because of this the foot will be forced to pronate. A pronating foot places abnormal stress on many areas of the foot, including the plantar fascia and the heel bone. This is how all of the heel problems noted above can start.

Chapter 7

Myofascial Pain Syndrome, Morton's Toe and Why You Can Hurt All Over

In Chapter 11, I will tell you about the remarkable life of Dr. Janet Travell, and her over fifty years of work regarding *Myofascial Pain Syndrome*. And, how it relates to Morton's Toe, and why it can make you feel miserable all over your body. The information about Myofascial Pain Syndrome in this chapter came mostly from a two-volume set of books by Dr. Travell's and Dr. David G. Simons called *Myofascial Pain and Dysfunction: the Trigger Point Manual*.[1] These books are acknowledged as the most important books ever written on this subject.

What is Myofascial Pain Syndrome?

First, don't be scared off by the long medical name. It is really pretty easy to understand. *Myofascial Pain Syndrome* are muscle pains. It can affect single muscles or groups of muscles, almost anywhere in your body. Myofascial Pain Syndrome can also cause you to be hurting at locations away from the painful muscle. This is called *referred pain*★. Dr. Travell wrote that it could also cause tenderness, muscle spasms, limitation of motion, depression, sleep disturbance and changes in circulation.[2]

How does Myofascial Pain Differ from Arthritis?

Most of the pains that are caused by Morton's Toe of the foot, ankle, knee, hip, and back are due to some form of arthritis. As I wrote before arthritis, are diseases of the joints and of the surrounding soft tissue structures of the joints. (i.e. bursas, capsules, tendons, and synovium). Arthritis and its associated soft tissue problems are not known for causing muscle pain or "referred pain" like Myofascial Pain Sydrome does. For our purposes, Myofascial pain is the pain that is caused by muscle dysfunction and the "referred pain" these muscles produce.

What Causes Myofascial Pain?

Besides Morton's Toe, which will be discussed next, there several other causes of Myofascial Pain Syndrome. These include:

1. mechanical stress, due to muscles that are just not working properly;
2. postural stresses, due to poor posture or sitting abnormally in bad chairs or desks
3. constriction of muscles, due to a tight stocking or a bag strap put over your shoulder for too long a time.

Myofascial Pain can also be caused by leg length discrepancies (one leg shorter than the other), vitamin deficiencies, slow metabolism, low blood sugar, depression, anxiety, infections, and sleep disorders.[3]

Morton's Toe and Myofascial Pain Sydrome

In her biography, Dr. Travell states how she was aware early in her career that when the second metatarsal bone was longer than the first metatarsal bone, it could transmit abnormal mechanical stress to the muscles of the ankle, knee, and hip joints that could result in having pain in these areas.[4]

As she wrote, "We [she and her father Dr. Willard Travell] had first learned about that congenital foot disorder, and how to correct it by padding the shoe, when Dr. Dudley J. Morton of Columbia University's Presbyterian Medical School discussed the subject before the Medical Society of the County of Kings, Section of Physical Therapy. The date was October 29, 1942, and it was a rainy night when my father and I drove out to Ocean Parkway in Brooklyn. I had a long day and Dr. Morton's lesson did not impress me then. My father drilled it into me."[5] Her father must have done a very good job of "drilling it into her" that evening because thereafter she recognized the problems of the first metatarsal bone, and the work of Dudley Morton, as an underlying, basic and significant cause of Myofascial Pain Syndrome. For the rest of her life she preferred using the term the "Dudley J. Morton's Foot" instead of Morton's Toe, but both are the same problems of the first metatarsal bone. Be it in her books with Dr. Simons, or in a 1990 videotape that she made, she explained and showed how and why the "Dudley J. Morton's Foot" (Morton's Toe) was one of the causes of Myofascial Pain Syndrome. By the way, Dr. Willard Travell (Janet's father) also was a big fan of Morton's work. He installed a cobbler table in his medical office, in order to re-mold patients' shoes as part of his treatment for their pains.[6]

How Morton's Toe Causes Myofascial Pain

In both of their books, Travell and Simons wrote a great deal about the "Dudley J. Morton's Foot" (Morton's Toe) and its relationship with Myofascial Pain Syndrome. This relationship is not hard to understand. If you have a Morton's Toe, your foot is not working right. This will cause many muscles to be stressed and injured. In Volume 2 of *Myofascial Pain & Dysfunction: The Trigger Point Manual,* the authors detail six muscles that can be activated or have "trigger points" due to the "Dudley Morton Foot." The amount of pain and suffering that can be caused by these six muscles is astounding. Here they are in what I feel is their order of importance in causing pain:

1. Gluteus Medius: this muscle can cause lower back pain (lumbago★), pain at the back and side of the buttock, and into the upper thigh (Fig. 7-1).[7]

2. Gluteus Minimus Muscle: the pain from this muscle can extend from the buttock down the thigh, knee, leg, calf and ankle.[8] Other doctors have stated that sciatic pain★ can be caused by this muscle (Fig. 7-2).[9]

3. Vastus Medialis Muscle: trigger points from this muscle can cause a referred pain on the front of the knee, and the lower thigh (Fig. 7-2).[10]

4. Peroneus Longus Muscle: referred pain from this muscle cause pain on the outside of the ankle and areas on the outside of the foot (Fig. 7-3).[11]

5. Posterior Tibial Muscle: the pains caused by this muscle start at the mid calf, goes over the Achilles tendon, over the heel and can cover the entire bottom of the foot and toes (Fig. 7-4).[12]

6. Flexor Digitorum Longus Muscle: this muscle causes pain mostly to the bottom of the middle of the fore-foot (Fig. 7-4).[13]

The bottom line is that pains of your back, thigh, knee, calf, leg, and of course pain in your ankles and feet can be due to Myofascial Pain, which in turn can be caused by having a Morton's Toe, or the "Dudley J. Morton's Foot." It can also cause *Temporomandibular Joint Pain* "TMJ" which is a problem that can make your teeth, jaw, cheek, eyes, eyebrows, and ears hurt. It can even cause headaches. According to Dr. Travell "TMJ" is a form of Myofascial Pain. In Chapter 12, I will write more about TMJ and Morton's Toe.

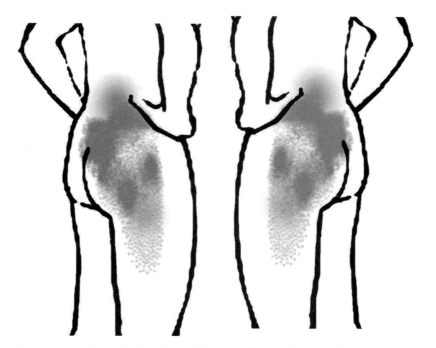

Fig. 7-1. According to Dr. Travell, the Gluteus Medius muscle is one of the muscles that can be affected by a Morton's Toe. The above diagrams show the places where you can have pain and trigger points of the lower back, the back, the side of the buttock, and the upper thigh from this muscle.

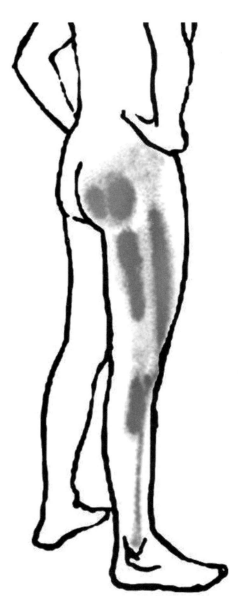

Fig. 7-2. This diagram shows the combined pain patterns and trigger points of two muscles: the Gluteus Minimus and the Vastus Medialis. Dr. Travell has stated that the Gluteus Minimus muscle can cause excruciating pain or trigger points starting at the buttock and going all the way down to the ankle, and including the thigh, the back of the knee, leg, and the calf. The Vastus Medialis muscle can cause pain at the front of the knee and the lower thigh. As before, Morton's Toe can trigger all of these pains.

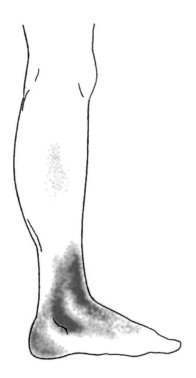

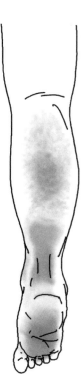

Fig. 7-3. The Peroneus Longus muscle causes pain on the outside of the ankle and outside of the foot.

Fig. 7-4. The pain patterns and trigger points caused by The Posterior Tibial and Flexor Digitorum Longus muscles are shown above. They can cause pain at the mid calf, Achilles tendon and bottom of mid-foot and toes.

The Videotapes

In 1990, Dr. Travell made a series of seven videotapes to educate health professionals about Myofascial Pain Syndrome. The tapes showed how to identify and treat those painful muscles throughout the body most often affected by myofascial pain. Of the seven tapes, only one was dedicated to a single subject. That tape was called "The Dudley J. Morton Foot" (Long Second Metatarsal).[14] Its purpose was to educate her fellow physicians regarding the important role the Morton's Toe can play in causing pain throughout the whole body.

It is hard to believe that Janet Travell was eighty-nine years old when she made this videotape. In it you see a highly intelligent and articulate physician delivering a lecture with an incredible ease and command of the facts concerning "The Dudley Morton Foot" and all the problems it can cause. To watch her hands, the same hands that treated two Presidents of the United States, craft her version of the pad to treat Morton's Toe is truly remarkable.

Fibromyalgia and Myofascial Pain

Like many other physicians I believe Myofascial Pain Syndrome and Fibromyalgia are very similar to one another. In my office, I refer to them as being "first cousins." They are both painful disorders of the muscles that affect millions, and makes their lives miserable. They are so similar that a medical textbook entitled *Myofascial Pain and Fibromyalgia* was written about the both of them.[15] Medical journals have also written about their similarities.[16] This is important because if you understand how a Morton's Toe can cause Myofascial Pain Syndrome, then you can understand why it can be the cause or part of the cause of why you may get fibromyalgia. I treat many women who have already been diagnosed with fibromyalgia. Many of them do have a Morton's Toe. Like those with Myofascial Pain Syndrome, many of these women with "Fibro" get better by applying a Toe Pad to their first metatarsal bone. If you have been diagnosed with Fibromyalgia, slowly try the Toe Pad to see if it helps. But be warned! The Toe Pad is very forceful and in fact can make someone with fibromyalgia worse. So the best thing to do is to try the Toe Pad only for about one or two hours a day for a week. If that feels good, then gradually add one hour every week, until your body gets used to the Toe Pad. Stop using the Toe Pad at once if it is hurting you. Regardless, the Toe Pad is not intended to cure Fibromyalgia. Its job is to stabilize the Morton's Toe so your "Fibro" will not get worse. I write more about Myofascial Pain Syndrome and Fibromyalgia in Chapter 12.

Dr. Janet Travell, one of the greatest physicians of the 20th century, has stated that if you have a Morton's Toe or the "Dudley J. Morton Foot" you could be prone to having pains throughout your whole body. Tell your friends and family. This is important stuff. If a loved one, a friend, or anyone you know has a chronic painful problem that no one, or no thing has helped, tell them to try the Toe Pad or other treatments I write about in the next chapter.

Chapter 8

The Toe Pad and Other Treatments for Morton's Toe

Throughout this book, I have written about the "Toe Pad". It is the term for the pad that I have used on thousands of patients during my career to treat the aches, pains, and torments caused by Morton's Toe. The truth is, the Toe Pad has nothing to do with the "Toe" but really is a pad that attaches to the bottom of the first metatarsal bone. It is much easier to say and write Toe Pad on a daily basis than saying the "first metatarsal bone pad." So that's why I have used the term Toe Pad all these years. The Toe Pad I use, and will show you how to make, is based on Dr. Morton's 1927 patented Compensating Insole Pad.[1] You can see Morton's original drawing for The Compensating Insole Pad beginning at page 219 of the Appendix.

Both the Toe Pad and Compensating Insole Pad accomplish the same thing. But after eighty years of use, the Toe Pad has become much smaller, and is easier to make than Morton's 1927 Compensating Insole Pad. The pads used by Dr. Janet Travell to treat her patients for the "Dudley Morton Foot" were also based on The Compensating Insole Pad but were also easier to make.[2]

How the Toe Pad Works to Make You Feel Better

According to Dr. Morton and Dr. Travell, if you have a short first metatarsal bone or hypermobility of the first metatarsal bone, it can cause excessive strain on the second metatarsal bone or other parts of your body and foot. It is this strain that can be the real cause of why you can be hurting not only of your foot, but also of your neck, back, hips, knees, legs and other places around your body.

The Toe Pad works by removing this strain, by acting as a platform on the bottom of the first metatarsal bone. This platform allows the first metatarsal bone to meet the ground properly and then forces it to bear weight normally. Once this happens, the abnormal strain that was improperly put on the second metatarsal bone to start with is removed and shifted back to the first metatarsal bone. It is this shifting of the abnormal strain off of the second metatarsal bone, back to the first metatarsal bone (where it belongs), that will start to have you feeling better again.[3]

The Toe Pad also acts as a platform in the treatment for Hypermobility of the First Metatarsal Bone. But now its job is to remove the slack of the ligaments in and around the bottom of the first metatarsal bone, which is causing excess motion of the bone. By doing this, the Toe Pad stabilizes and also locks the first metatarsal bone in place.[4] Once the bone is locked in place, it will help control all of the problems not only of the feet, but also throughout the body associated with Hypermobility of the First Metatarsal Bone.[5]

What You Need to Make the Toe Pad

The materials you need to make the Toe Pad are easy to find. There is nothing special about them, and most probably, you already have many of them. But first allow me to tell you another true story to show you that you can use almost anything in making the Toe Pad.

Many years ago, sometime in the 1970s, before I fully understood the importance of the Morton's Toe, and how it worked, the following events indeed took place to me.

One day in a bar, I struck up a conversation with an older man. After talking for a while, I mentioned to him that I was a foot doctor. He said he had very bad feet for some time but kept them pain-free for years by doing something unusual. Well, of course I was interested, and then asked him to tell me what he did.

Well, he said, "I slip off the whole cellophane wrapping of two packs of Winston cigarettes, fold them in half and tape it right behind my big toe, and my pain stays away from my foot for about 3–4 days. One pack is not enough and three packs are too much, no, exactly the wrapping from two packs works."

I looked at him in disbelief, and then said, "Cellophane wrapping from two packets of Winstons?" "Yep, two packs," he said.

The points of this true story are:

a. you can use almost "anything" to get the first metatarsal bone lifted up

b. it does not take much of this "anything" to do it

Remember, for a good part of the 20th century, treating foot pain by lifting the first metatarsal bone was common knowledge. It might be new news to a lot of people today, but it was not years ago.

Materials I Like

The aim of the Toe Pad is to lift the first metatarsal bone. As shown above, almost anything that does that is fine. But here are some simple things I like.

Spongy foam is a great material for making the Toe Pad. The easiest place to get the foam is to cut up a pair of those cheap cushioned shoe insoles.

You have seen the cushioned shoe insoles before. They are those flimsy things you put into your shoes. They come in cellophane packs (Fig. 8-1). Their advantages are that they are cheap and easy to get. They sell them all over, in supermarkets, chain stores, Wal-Mart, Kmart and discount stores. A pair of these insoles should cost about $1.69 to $1.99. I saw some no-name brands for under $1.00, even better. You will need to buy at least 2 packs of the insoles. I will explain why shortly. In a moment, I will explain how you cut the insoles up to use the spongy foam.

Besides the foam from the shoe insole, I have found that Dr. Scholl's Molefoam® is a good material in making the Toe Pad. The nice things about the Molefoam are that it has an adhesive backing and is a little easier to use. Most stores should have it in their foot products departments, but if you cannot find it, there it is readily available on the Internet for $3.00–5.00 a pack. One pack should keep you comfortable for several weeks. If you cannot get the Molefoam®, any type of Moleskin with an adhesive backing should also work.

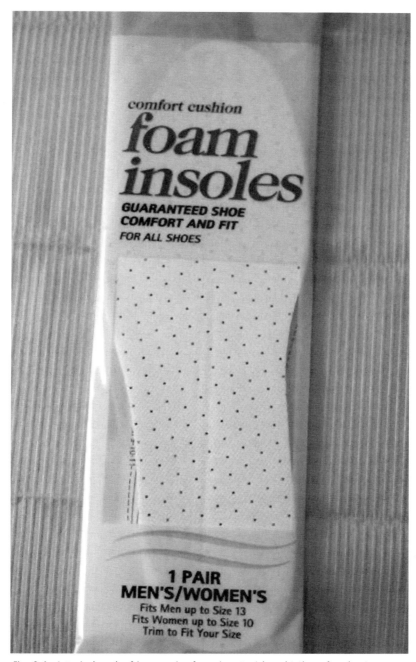

Fig. 8-1. A typical pack of inexpensive foam inserts. I bought these for about $1.00 at a local store. It is a good idea to buy two or three packs of these.

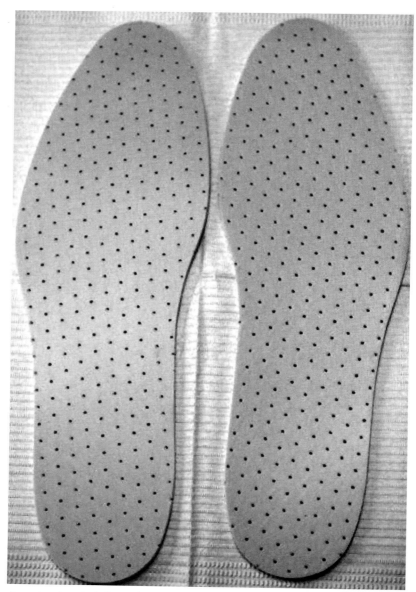

Foam inserts out of the pack.

Many other materials that you can find around your home like cork, felt, foam, plastic, cardboard and sponge can also be used in making the Toe Pad. As I said above, in the end it really does not matter what type of material that you use, as long as it lifts the first metatarsal bone just a little. Remember our friend with the two cellophane wrappings from the Winstons.

Making The Toe Pad

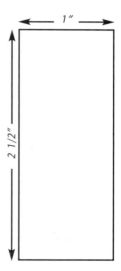

Once you have picked the material you want to use, this is how you make the Toe Pad. Look at this drawing:

Now to start with, just cut a piece of your material to about the size of the drawing.

Later on, depending on your size, you may need to make it shorter or longer. But for now, just cut it to about the size of this drawing – about 1" by 2 1/2". It doesn't have to be exact or pretty.

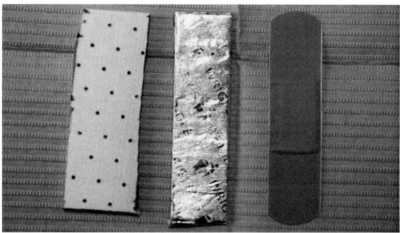

Fig. 8-2. The Toe Pad is about the same size as a stick of chewing gum or a Band-Aid®.

If you have any doubts just make it the size of a stick of gum, or a Bandaid® (Fig. 8-2).

Great! You have just made your first Toe Pad. Now make two more just like it. You are now ready to attach the Toe Pad to the bottom of your first metatarsal bone.

Putting the Toe Pad on your Foot, or Finding the Head of the First Metatarsal Bone

This is not hard to do. Look at the photo below to help you. Look at the bottom of your foot. Now, pull your toes up toward you. Right below where the big toe attaches to the foot you will see a bulge.

This bulge is the head of the first metatarsal bone (Fig. 8-3).

Put one end of the Toe Pad directly over the bulge (first metatarsal head) with the rest of the Toe Pad (the

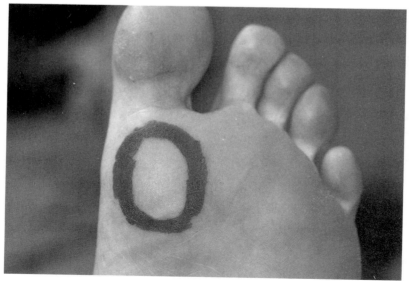

Fig. 8-3. Circled head of first metatarsal bone.

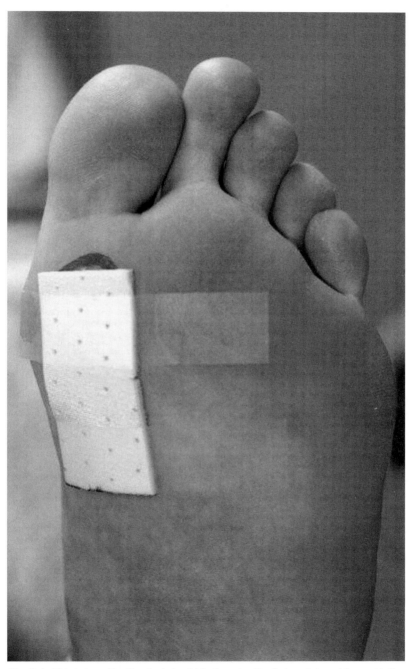

Fig. 8-4. This is how the Toe Pad should look under the first metatarsal bone. Notice how it goes up and down.

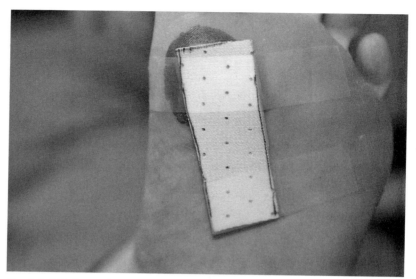

Fig. 8-5. This Toe Pad is misaligned, and not lying right along the first metatarsal bone. It should be running straight up and down.

long part) pointed straight down, going away from the bulge. It is easy. Just look at Fig. 8-4 and copy that. Just be sure the Toe Pad is not pointed toward the inside part of the foot but is lying right next to the edge of the foot

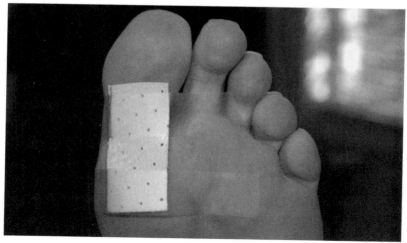

Fig. 8-6. This pad is also not right. It should not be going this far up to the big toe.

(Fig. 8-5). The top of the pad should not go beyond the bulge of the first metatarsal head. Make sure it never goes past the first metatarsal head toward the bottom of the big toe (Fig. 8-6).

Once you get the pad lined up right, you can then attach it to the bottom of the foot as follows.

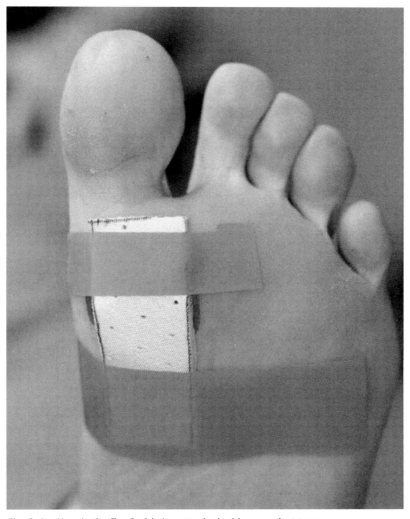

Fig. 8-6a. Here is the Toe Pad being attached with some duct tape.

1. If the Toe Pad has adhesive backing, just remove the paper backing, and stick it to the bottom of the first metatarsal bone as I just described.

2. If your Toe Pad does not have adhesive backing, attach it to the bottom of the first metatarsal bone with anything you may have that can make it stick. To start with, it doesn't matter what you use to make it stick or what it looks like. Athletic tape, duct tape (Fig. 8-6a), scotch tape, electrical tape, glue, band-aids, or rubber bands are just some of the possible things you can use. All that I care about, to start with, is getting your Toe Pad to make contact and stick (just a little) to the bottom of the first metatarsal bone. Now, stand up, without your sock.

Congratulations! You have just changed the way your foot and maybe your whole body works. The Toe Pad will make you feel a little different, but hopefully better. You can take the Toe Pad off when you sleep or shower.

At all times, make sure the pad does not shift and is still lying correctly on the foot.

Depending on your size, you may need to make the Toe Pad longer or shorter to feel good for you. That's okay. There is no right or wrong. I encourage you to experiment to find the length of the pad that works the best for you.

How to Put Your Socks or Hose On

Not everyone wears socks. But if you do, this is how you put them on while wearing the Toe Pad. Take the sock and roll it up like a little cap (Fig. 8-7). Then, slowly

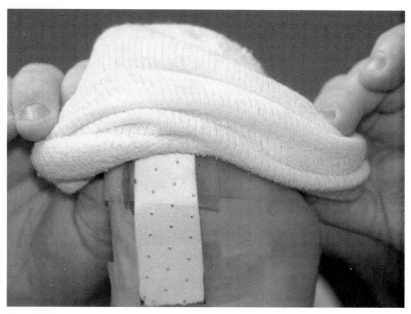

Fig. 8-7. Putting socks on properly over Toe Pad. Roll it up like a little cap and work it over the toes.

work it down over your foot. Do not drag or pull it on because it can cause the Toe Pad to move or roll up.

You May Need to Add More Layers to the Toe Pad

When you first start wearing the Toe Pad, you may need to make it thicker depending on your size and weight. This is simple to do. Just stack (like pancakes) one Toe Pad on top of another Toe Pad until you have the number of layers that makes you feel good (Fig. 8-8). You may need to experiment to see what is best for you. You attach these layers of Toe Pad to one another the same way you put the Toe Pad on your first metatarsal bone. If the Toe Pad has adhesive backing, just take the paper backing off and attach them to one another. If the Toe

Pad you are using does not have an adhesive back, put them together using any one of the ways I suggested above. There is no problem in just scotch taping 2 or 3 layers together (Fig. 8-9).

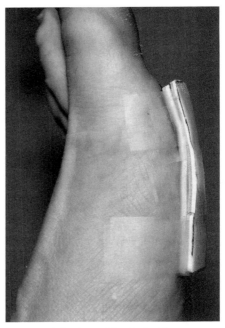

Once that is done, stick the Toe Pad back on the bottom of the first metatarsal bone. I don't care what it looks like right now. All I care about is that you might be starting to feel better.

Fig. 8-8. Side view of Toe Pad with two layers of material taped together.

It is not unusual to start to feel better from wearing the Toe Pad, only to have the pains return after several days. This is very common because the Toe Pad become flattened down from your wearing it, and is now no longer as thick as it needs to be. Remember, the two packs of Winstons had to be changed every 3-4 days. Well, you may have to do that with the Toe Pad to start with. No problem, all we need to do is fatten the Toe Pad up again. Simply put a new layer of material on top of the previous layers. After doing this a couple of times, the pad will become thick enough on its own so it won't flatten out and be a problem.

Finally, our humble little Toe Pad is really a very dynamic device that will cause your foot and body to work differently for the first time in years. Because of

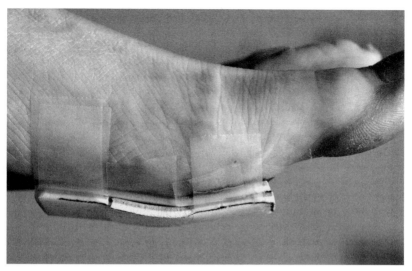

Fig. 8-9. Another view of a doubled layered Toe Pad.

this, you may get new discomforts in places on your body that you never had before. Pains at the back, knee, hip and legs are not uncommon in some people. But these new pains will shortly disappear once your body gets adjusted to working normally with the Toe Pad. If, after several days, these new discomforts are not improved, take the Toe Pad off and don't wear it until you feel better. Then start over with a thinner pad.

If you have a lot of long-standing arthritis in your body, or fibromyalgia **be very careful.** Only wear the Toe Pad for a few hours a day for a week or so, until your body/joints get used to these new changes. If you wear it too much too soon, you might be hurting a lot. If this happens, stop wearing it until you feel better. Then, try a thinner pad for fewer hours.

Your New Best Friend May Be George Washington

If you are hurting and not able to get to the store to buy the material needed, or cannot find anything at home to make a Toe Pad, there is a short-term fix that you can use. Take a quarter, a 25-cent piece, and tape it under your first metatarsal head. A couple of pieces of scotch tape is all you need (Fig. 8-10).

This is not as a good as the Toe Pad, but for a short period of a time it can treat the aches and pains caused by Morton's Toe pretty well. I have used this many times when I was out of my office and needed to help someone. The quarter lifts the first metatarsal head just enough to make a difference. But as soon as possible, go to the Toe Pad for relief.

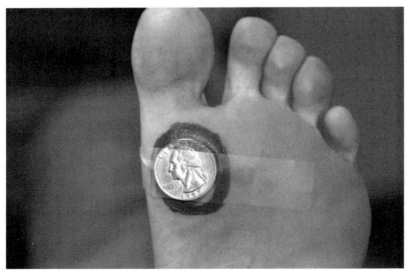

Fig. 8-10. A 25 cent piece taped to the bottom of the first metatarsal head to be a short term fix to treat a Morton's Toe.

The Shoe Insert

Once you have worn the Toe Pad for a while, you may want to try the Shoe Insert. The Shoe Insert is nothing more than the Toe Pad attached to something like a cushioned insole. The big advantage with the Shoe Insert is that because it is changeable from shoe to shoe you won't have to take the Toe Pad on and off your skin everyday. This will make your life a lot easier.

The Shoe Inserts are also cheap to make. In no way should a pair cost more than a few dollars. All that you need are two pairs of the cheap foam insoles to make them.

How to Make the Shoe Insert

The Shoe Insert is made up of two parts: the Base and our old friend, the Toe Pad.

The Base: The purpose of the Base is to serve as a place to which the Toe Pad can park itself other than attaching directly on to the skin, at the bottom of the first metatarsal bone. Remember, I told you to buy two pairs of the cheap cushioned shoe insoles. The first pair you may have used in making the Toe Pad. Well, the second pair will be the base of the Shoe Insert. All that you need to do is to take the cushioned shoe insoles from the cellophane package and trim them so the whole insole fits into your shoes (Fig. 8-11).

Another thing you can use for the base of the Shoe Insert is one of those removable thin inserts that came inside your tennis shoes and other types of shoes.

Most of the time they are not glued down, so they can easily be pulled out. Even if they are glued down, they are

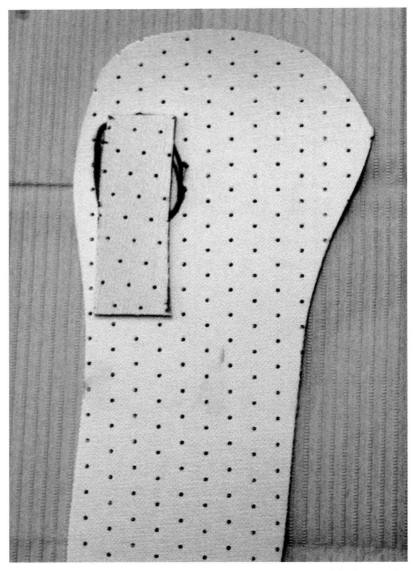

Fig. 8-11. This is the "Shoe Insert." Notice how Toe Pad is on top of the base, right under the first metatarsal bone.

really doing nothing to help your feet. So you might as well pull them out of those shoes and use them as the base for your Shoe Inserts and save a couple of dollars.

Don't waste your money on arch supports, as they won't work for this. All that you need is the cheap foam insole or the insert from your shoe and sneaker. Your problem is not your arch but near the ball of your foot. I will discuss arch supports later in Chapter 14.

The Toe Pad: This is the same pad that you made and attached to the bottom of your foot, at the first metatarsal bone. In the Shoe Insert, the Toe Pad will attach on to the base. Go ahead and prepare two new Toe Pads as you did before. But instead of putting them on your foot, set them aside for now. You will use them shortly.

How to Put the Toe Pad and Base Together to Make the Shoe Insert

With your socks off do the following:
1. Put the trimmed foam insole (base) into your shoe.
2. As you did earlier, locate on the bottom of your foot, the bulge that is the head of the first metatarsal bone (Fig. 8-3).
3. With a lipstick or a marker, make a heavy mark at the bulge at the first metatarsal head on the bottom of your foot (see Fig. 8-3). This is the same spot where you first attached the Toe Pad to your foot.
4. Put your shoe back on without your sock and rock back and forth on the ball of your foot for a moment.
5. Take your shoe off, remove the insole, and find the spot made by the lipstick or marker left on the cushioned

shoe insole. It may be very faint, but if found, circle it with a pen or marker.

6. If this doesn't work, just wear the foam shoe insole in your shoe for 2–3 days and the depression under the head of first metatarsal bone should then appear.

Attaching the Toe Pad to the Base

The Toe Pad attaches to the base the same way it attached to the skin on the bottom of the first metatarsal bone. Do the following:

1. Find the circle or mark on the top side of the base that you made. This mark is the head of the first metatarsal bone.

2. Now, as you did on your foot, place one end of the Toe Pad directly over the circle, or mark, on the top of the base at the first metatarsal head. Then line up the Toe Pad along the top of the base going straight down—away from the mark. This is exactly how you lined up the Toe Pad on the bottom of the first metatarsal bone, except now you are doing it on the top of the base.

   Once lined up, attach the Toe Pad to the base, with tape, glue or anything else that works for you (Fig. 8-11).

3. In the alternative, find the area on the bottom side of the base which is directly under that circled or marked area, and attach the pad onto the bottom side of the foam insole, the same way it would have been attached on the top.

4. It doesn't matter if the Toe Pad is on the top or bottom of the base. Use the one which you are more comfortable with.

5. Gently return the base, with the Toe Pad attached, back into your shoe.

6. Put your shoes on with socks; be careful not to roll or crease it, especially if the Toe Pad is attached to the top of the base. Okay, let's take your Shoe Inserts for a test drive.

7. As when the pad was on your skin, you may need to reposition the location of the Toe Pad on the base for the Shoe Insert to feel good. After wearing the Shoe Insert for several days, you may notice that your feet and body bother you again for no apparent reason. Like before, when the pad was directly on your foot, it can flatten down. All that you will need to do is to add a new layer to the preexisting Toe Pad. By doing this, you are building up the Toe Pad to find its proper thickness.

In the beginning of treating their Morton's Toe, many people tell me that it is easier for them just to apply the Toe Pad directly to the bottom of their metatarsal bone just to get the feel of it. But eventually, most people gravitate toward the Shoe Inserts because there is less wear and tear on the skin, and in general, the Shoe Insert is easier to use. If you like the Shoe Insert you can then make it for each pair of your shoes. If you get tired of doing this and want something more permanent, you can go see your podiatrist and get an orthotic (next chapter) custom-made for your foot.

Treatment for Heels

For the most part, Plantar Fasciitis, Heel Bursitis, Heel Spurs, and other common heel problems can get better by using the Toe Pad or Shoe Inserts. But, because the arch and heel take more stress and strain than any other parts of the foot, they may need some extra help to control the morning pains and other distress you are having. I suggest you start out with the Toe Pad or Shoe Inserts and see how your arch and/or heel problems respond to it. If, after several days you find there is no improvement, make the following change.

The Heel Addition

The purpose of the heel addition is to work in combination with the Toe Pad to form a unit to take the maximum strain off of the arch and heel. It has proven to be awesome in reducing the pain in this area. You can put it directly on your foot, or make it part of a Shoe Insert. The foam from the foam insoles or other materials can be used to make the heel addition, but you may need several layers of it to make it thick enough. The size of the heel addition is like a half oval. Cut it to the following template (Fig. 8-12).

Or, you can also make the heel addition by cutting off the bottom section of a foam insole (Fig. 8-13).

Again, make it larger or smaller depending on your size. Look at Fig. 8-14 to see how the heel addition and the Toe Pad come together on your foot or on the Shoe Insert. Ideally, the end of the Toe Pad and the end of the heel addition are touching or "kissing" each other. This is important because it is this butting together of the Toe

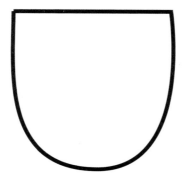

Fig. 8-12. This is the size of the heel addition that you can cut out of almost any material.

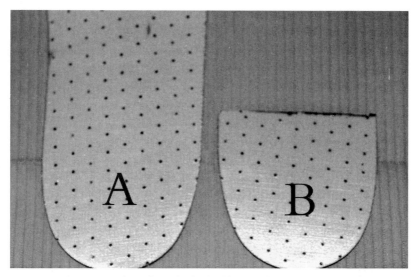

Fig. 8-13. This picture shows how the heel addition "B" can be cut/made from the bottom of the foam insole "A".

Pad and heel addition that makes it such a dynamic unit.

The major caution with the heel addition is to make sure you don't put it too far down the foot, toward the heel because it might cut into the heel area and cause discomfort. Make sure the heel addition is not touching the heel. Again, experiment with it, and you will see putting it

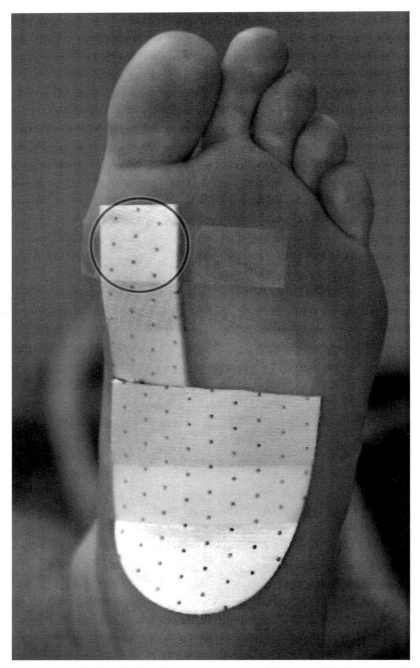

Fig. 8-14. Toe Pad and heel addition on the bottom of the foot. Circled area is head of the first metatarsal bone.

squarely under the arch should make it work fine. Please note, this is not an arch support. The Toe Pad, in combination with the heel addition, is what makes this work. No arch support can compete with the good medicine that this pad is based on.

No treatment works for everyone; this includes the Toe Pad, Shoe Inserts and heel addition. If, after a reasonable time, you are still hurting with a foot, arch or heel problem, I would absolutely encourage you to seek professional care for these podiatric ailments.

Chapter 9

Other Treatments for Morton's Toe – Self Care

Banging Your Hand

Close your eyes and imagine that for some strange reason, you have been banging your hand against a wall, every day, for thirty years. You do not know why, but you just keep banging away at that hand. In spite of the fact your hand is now red, swollen, throbbing, and aching you just keep banging and banging and banging away. One day a light bulb goes on in your head and commands you to "Stop banging youy hand", so you finally stop. Great! No more banging of your hand! But now what? Well, your hand won't get any worse, assuming you don't go back to banging it. But thanks to thirty years of banging your hand, your hand is still very damaged. Remember that redness, swelling, throbbing and aching? Well, it is still there and hasn't left. And, it's not going to be healed overnight. No, it is going to take some time to repair the injury that you have inflicted on your poor little hand, and you will need some form of treatment to help heal it.

Now, open your eyes, and discover what I was really writing about. I was not really writing about your hand, but was really writing about your feet. The same damage that I described about your hand is exactly what has happened to your feet, over a period of time. Except, it is worse to your feet because you don't walk on your hands. That sounds stupid, but it is true. If your hand was hurt, you can stop using it. You do not have that luxury with your feet, unless you can get completely off of them or have a couple of big guys carry you around the whole day.

The Toe Pad and/or Shoe Inserts should start to help you and stop your feet from getting any worse, as long as you wear them. But that is only part of the treatment in getting you back to normal. Just like the hand, after all those years of banging your feet against the ground, there is an abnormal build-up of redness, swelling, throbbing and aching. The good news is there are many simple things you can do at home to heal your long damaged feet.

Home Treatments to Help Your Feet and Body

Heat

I love heat for the treatment of chronic foot problems. Some people may disagree with me, and say ice is better. Ice is okay right after an injury, like when you twist your ankle. Besides that, heat is the best way to go, for you to mend your own damaged feet.

Why Heat?

The most obvious reason is the wonderful soothing effect heat has. It will just make you feel better. This is for the simple reason that heat will increase the blood flowing into the foot. When more blood is brought into the foot, it will start to remove all of the damaged tissues that has built up over a period of years. This buildup was due to the constant abuses that your feet were exposed to. Once you start to flush, or push out this stuff, the redness, swelling, throbbing and aching in your feet and other parts of your body will start to go away.

How It Works

The best way I can explain this is to tell you about the puddle versus the water hose. If you have a large puddle of water that was caused by a heavy rain in front of your house, you might want to get rid of it. So how do you do it? Well, you can take a bucket and with several trips get rid of it that way. Or you can take a broom and sweep it away. Or, you can take your hose and by using the sprayer, push more water into the puddle, making it wash away. That is exactly what you are doing with soaks, heating pads, and a paraffin bath (see below). You are washing away, and pushing out, the abnormal buildup of inflammation due to injuries by draining more blood into the damaged area.

Podiatrists have understood this concept for years, and often will give a nerve block in the foot in order to increase the circulation. When certain nerves in the foot are numbed or blocked, it has the effect of causing the blood vessels to open up wider and bring more blood down into the foot. This increase in blood flow decreases pain and inflammation by washing away all of the rubbish that has built up over time in your foot. Basically, this is the same concept as the hose and the puddle. And, this is what you will be doing when you use heat to bring more blood into your feet.

Right now, I can hear someone saying, "Dr. Schuler, I soaked my feet daily and it only gave me temporary relief in the past." My answer to that statement is "ABSOLUTELY!"

Of course, it only gave you temporary relief because every time you stood up after soaking, you were immediately re-injuring your feet. Now you are hopefully treating the foot by using the Toe Pad or Shoe Insert. By doing this, you will limit or even stop your feet from being re-damaged every time you walk. When combined with daily heat treatments, you will be addressing both reasons why your feet and body may have been hurting and hopefully you should start to get better.

Heating Pads, Paraffin Baths and Soaks

I have found that most people at home can use heating pads, paraffin baths, or soaks. Regardless of which one you use, the aim is to decrease your pain by increasing blood flow to the damaged areas of your feet. This is the key to your healing. The trick is to use them on a daily basis, several times a day if you can.

Before you use any of them, be sure to read the FDA guidelines starting on page 120.

Heating Pads

Common sense demands that you do not make the heating pad too hot. It you have any difficulties in feeling the proper temperature due to any type of problem, you may have to use your elbow to feel the warmth of the pad or get someone to check it for you. Moreover, if you have any doubts get the permission of your own physician before you start.

Paraffin Baths

One of my favorite home heat treatments is a paraffin bath. It is one of the most effective methods of applying deep heat to relieve pain and stiffness. A paraffin bath is a plastic tub in which you melt wax. You dip your foot into the tub of wax,

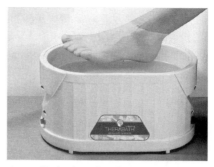

A paraffin bath with a foot about to be dipped into it. (Courtesy WR Medical Electronics Co.)

applying several coats of wax up to the level of the ankle. Then you wrap your feet up in towels. The hot wax then sends great amounts of blood down to your feet. It is also great for painful hands. A good one costs about $150, but I saw one last year at Wal-Mart for about $50. With regular use, it can help remove the chronic pain, swelling, soreness, aching, and throbbing from your feet and ankles. As above, before using a paraffin bath, make sure there is no medical reason why you shouldn't.

Soaks

Since the time that man has been hanging out in caves, we have been sticking our bodies in warm water to feel better. Be it a pan of water, a warm tub, or a trip to your spa: soaking parts of our body has always been a neat thing to do. From the standpoint of our feet, soaking will flush your feet by bringing blood to it. As I said previously, this flushing will heal our feet by washing away damaged tissues that have collected over a period of time. By getting this junk out of the injured areas in your feet, you will start to feel better.

DO NOT make the water very hot – warm is just fine. Do not waste any money by putting anything in the water unless you want to. What is important is that you soak your feet several times a day for about twenty minutes, if you can... assuming there are no contraindications to do so.

I am so concerned with this that please find reprinted below the Food and Drugs Administration booklet on the proper use of heating devices.

PLEASE READ BEFORE USING ANY HEATING DEVICE INCLUDING THE HEATING PAD OR PARAFFIN BATH.

HEATING DEVICES – HOW TO AVOID BURNS
BY JOAN FERLO TODD, RN, BSN, Nurse Consultant, Food and Drug Administration Center for Devices and Radiological Health, Rockville, MD.

A PATIENT WITH ARTHRITIS SUFFERED A SECOND DEGREE BURN to the hip after receiving treatment with a heating pad for pain. Set at low, the heating pad was left on for less than 20 minutes with the patient lying on top of the pad. Later testing showed that the pad was working properly and met the manufacturer's specifications. What went wrong? Therapeutic heating devices, such as heating pads, hot packs, and hot water bottles, although generally safe, can cause burns. Most burns result from improper use or use with inappropriate patients, such as infants and elderly patients. The severity of the burn is influenced by factors such as heat intensity, length of application, and the patient's age, medical history, and ability to sense pain. What precautions can you take?

Follow these do's and don'ts to keep your patient safe when using heating devices:

- DO inspect the device before each use to ensure it's in proper condition.

- DO read directions and contraindications for use.

- DO use a protective cover.

- DO place the pad or pack on top of not underneath the patient.

- DO assess skin integrity frequently and adjust the therapy interval according to the patient's skin tolerance – no longer than 15 to 20 minutes.

- DON'T use the device on someone who's sleeping or unconscious, an infant, or a patient with altered mental status or decreased skin sensation (such as people with diabetes or compromised skin circulation).

- DON'T use pins to fasten the device in place.

- DON'T use with ointments or salve preparations containing heat-producing ingredients.

- DON'T use electrical heating devices in an oxygen-enriched environment or near oxygen-emitting equipment.

Most of the above is common sense but it was important that you read it.

If after using the home heat treatments for a while in combination with the Toe Pad, you are still hurting more than you want to, it is time to see your friendly, local foot specialist. Please don't suffer with foot pains. Just because my suggestions did not work does not mean you cannot be helped.

Orthotics

I hope the Toe Pad and/or Shoe Insert will help your foot problems and any other problems that are caused by your Morton's Toe. However, as I stated back on page 17, besides Morton's Toe, there are many other actions, stress, strains and forces that can cause the foot and body to hurt. If you want to address these other problems and can afford it, you need to have custom-made orthotics fabricated for yourself.

What are Orthotics?

In laymen's terms, orthotics are custom-made Shoe Inserts that are used to make a foot that is not working properly, work properly.

Orthotics may look like "arch supports," but other than them both going inside your shoes, they have nothing in common.

The job of orthotics is not only to address the problems caused by the Morton's Toe, but also help control

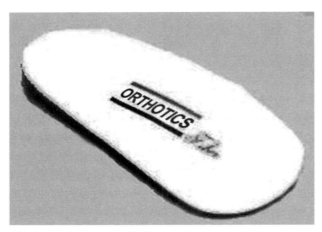

This is a custom-made orthotic.

the other defects that are affecting your foot and body when you are standing, walking, and running. Orthotics will keep you out of pain by controlling these problems in your foot. There are different types of orthotics. Depending on your problems, your podiatrist or other licensed health professional will determine which type is best for you.

How Orthotics Work

Orthotics work in the same way that eyeglasses work. Glasses make it possible for you to see better immediately by removing the stress, strain and overload from the eyes, as long as you are wearing them. But the second you take the glasses off, you are left with the same old eyeballs that don't work right. Glasses do not cure, but accommodate★ your eye problems. That is exactly what orthotics do for the foot. They don't cure, they accommodate. Stop wearing the orthotics and all of the abnormal problems your foot had in the past will come back. The same goes for the Toe Pad or Shoe Insert. Let me explain it another way. If you have a bad cough that is caused by an infection you not only need a cough syrup to stop the cough, but you will need an antibiotic to kill off the germs that caused the cough. If you don't get the antibiotic, the cough might not ever totally go away. That is the same exact situation with orthotics. You could have the best foot surgery ever done in the history of the world, only to see the same problem return because you did not get orthotics to control the real problem of your feet not working right. Sorry, orthotics are not a cure! That is okay, because they might as well be as long as you wear them.

How Orthotics are Made

A properly crafted orthotic is made under the direction of a podiatrist, or another trained, licensed health care professional. First, an examination is done with or without X-rays, and then an impression (cast) of the feet is mostly likely made. The purpose of taking the impression, and the secret of making a properly made orthotic, is to capture a true anatomical position★ (copy) of the foot. This is essential in so that the proper positions and adjustments can be built into the orthotic in order for it to work properly. Taking the impression is an art that takes some experience to learn properly. I have always made my impressions of the feet in the most classical way, with plaster of paris. This is called a slipper cast.

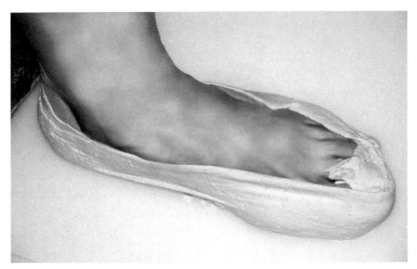

A slipper cast.

Another acceptable technique used by many doctors to capture the proper position of the foot when making the orthotic is to have the patient step down into a Styrofoam-lined box.

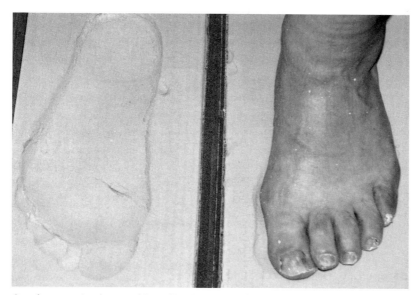

Styrofoam casting box used for taking impression for foot orthotics.

A newer technique used by some podiatrists is a computer mat that the patient walks across. This also gives the podiatrist the facts they need in making the orthotics. Any of these three methods is acceptable in getting the proper information, assuming it is done by a properly trained professional. The custom-made slipper cast impression, Styrofoam-lined box, or computer information is then sent to a laboratory where the orthotic will be fabricated to meet the unique needs of the patient.

Arch supports, bought in an arch support store regardless of the price, can never accomplish this. In Chapter 15, I will write a lot more about arch supports.

Surgery

In the early part of my career, I performed a great deal of foot surgery. As stated before, I wrote a book about it in the early 1980s. I still perform foot surgery when needed, but now thanks to Dr. Morton, I do much fewer foot surgeries for such problems as corns, callouses, burning feet, bunions, hammer toes or heel pains. If you are truly in need of foot surgery, by all means, have it done. However, before having the surgery, ask your doctor if you have a Morton's Toe or other orthopedic foot problems. If the answer is "yes," ask him or her about treating the Morton's Toe first. You

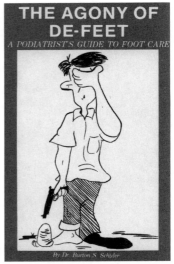

Cover of Dr. Schuler's 1982 book "The Agony of De-Feet A Podiatrist's Guide to Foot Care."

may very likely find that your pains will go away and there will be no need for surgery, after treating the Morton's Toe. If it turns out you still need the foot surgery, you have lost nothing in treating the Morton's Toe. The reason for this is that any foot surgery performed has a much greater chance of success if the abnormal forces caused by the Morton's Toe are treated and under control. It is a "no-lose" situation for both you and the doctor to treat the problems caused by the Morton's Toe before any foot surgery. But, if your doctor honestly states that they just don't know about Morton's Toe, that is okay, but encourage them to buy this book.

Cures

I try hard never to use the words 'guarantee' or 'cure' in my office. Nothing works 100% of the time. Having a foot surgery is not a cure. Be it for a bunion, a hammer toe, a neuroma, a corn, callus, or heel spur; you are not being cured! All that the surgery is doing is getting rid of the problem you came in with. As I stated above, the closest thing to a cure is getting an orthotic. Until you control the abnormal stress of the abnormal foot by getting an orthotic, nothing has really changed. You can end up back where you started with the same problem again. If you're dedicating the time, expense, pain and inconvenience of having a foot surgery, invest the extra money and allow your podiatrist to fabricate custom orthotics for you. They are well worth it.

Chapter 10

Dr. Dudley Joy Morton

I n the first half of the twentieth century, the most famous doctor in the United States, regarding problems of the human foot, was Dudley J. Morton, M.D. During that time, such publications as *Readers Digest,*[1] *Time Magazine,*[2] and *The New York Times*[3] regularly quoted and cited him. He was repeatedly written

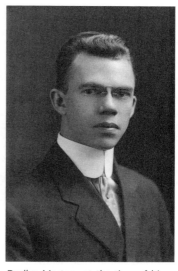

Dudley Morton, at the time of his medicial school graduation, 1907 (courtesy Morton Family).

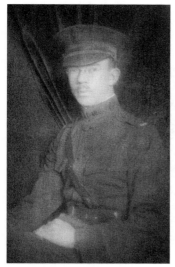

Dr. Morton during World War I (courtesy Morton Family).

about in dozens of newspapers around the country. His medical books and articles on the foot were the leading authorities of their time.

Aside from being a renowned authority of the foot, Morton was also an orthopedic surgeon, anatomist, evolutionist, teacher, anthropologist, author, musician, painter and inventor. He was born on March 27, 1884 in Baltimore, Maryland, on his family's farm. In 1907, Morton graduated from Hahemann Medical College in Pennsylvania.

During World War I, he went to France and served as a surgeon with the famous American Ambulance of Paris.[4]

When he returned from the war, Dr. Morton became a research associate at the American Museum of Natural History in New York, where he served as an anatomist. While at the museum, he concerned himself with the evolutionary development of the human foot. This is where he started to establish his reputation. His numerous papers and studies in the early and mid-1920s revolved around his study of primates (monkeys). This laid the groundwork for his most important work pertaining to the human foot, which took place in the late 1920s. In Chapter 14, I will tell you much more about this work.

Besides his scientific publications, in 1924, he found the time to write and publish a delightful children's book called "The Grampa's Toy Shop."[5] This delightful, highly imaginary Christmas story shows how diverse and creative Dr. Morton truly was.

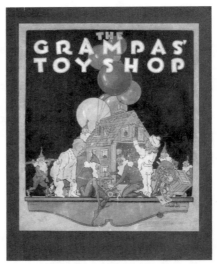

Cover of Dr. Morton's children book, The Grampas' Toy Shop.

Two Important Papers

Between 1924 and 1928, Morton was on the faculty of the Yale University School of Medicine where he was an assistant professor in the Department of Surgery. While at Yale, he published the two papers that would present, for the first time, what Morton's Toe was. In 1927, he published his first paper in the prestigious *Journal of Bone and Joint Surgery* titled "Metatarus Atavicu: The Identification of a Distinctive Type of Foot Disorder."[6] This scientific paper was the first time Morton presented his theory of the short first metatarsal bone and the harmful effects it could cause on the foot.

The following year, in 1928, Morton published another paper in the *Journal of Bone and Joint Surgery.* This paper described, for the first time, another condition of the first metatarsal bone known as "Hypermobility of the First Metatarsal Bone."[7] This condition and the short first metatarsal bone are the two inherited foot problems that compose Morton's Toe. (Dr. Morton never referred to these two problems as a Morton's Toe. This is the term that was given to these problems over a period of time by the medical profession.)

As I wrote previously, these two problems are responsible for alot of the suffering, not only of the foot but throughout the body.

The Insole or Toe Pad

In his 1927 paper, Dr. Morton described a pad-insole he invented to treat the problems caused by the improperly working short first metatarsal bone. Realizing this device was new, different and literally one of a kind, Dudley

Morton did a very, very smart thing. On June 20, 1927, he applied for a patent on his insole, which he called "Means for Compensating for Foot Abnormalities." It took almost five years, but on March 1, 1932, Dudley J. Morton was granted U.S. Patent # 1,847,973 for his device. (See page 219 to take a look at the patent application.) The Toe Pad/Shoe Insole, which I described in this book, is based on Morton's 1927 patented device. After over eighty years, its basic concept is still the best way of treating the problems of the foot and body associated with Morton's Toe.

Books

If the 1920s was Morton's decade of writing scientific articles, the 1930s through 1950s was his era of writing books, both for the medical community and the general public. During those years, he wrote seven books. As before, these books were about evolution, anatomy, and the human foot. In 1934, 1941, and 1944, he wrote three books on anatomy and disection.

The Human Foot

The most important of his books was the *The Human Foot* (1935) – the one I paid eight bucks for. It was written as a textbook for the medical community. The basis of the book came directly from his 1927 and 1928 papers written for the *Journal of Bone and Joint Surgery* in conjunction with his years of research as an anatomist, anthropologist, and evolutionist. His years of work at the American Museum of National History, Yale, and Columbia were also reflected in the book. In *The Human Foot,* Morton laid out, step-by-step, via evolution and inheritances, why we have foot problems and what to do about them. He explains (as noted previously) that the two major causes of foot problems were the short first metatarsal bone and hypermobility of the first metatarsal bone. In spite of the fact that over eighty years have passed, the material Morton presented in *The Human Foot* is still true. Not only to those suffering with foot problems, but as you have seen, for those who also suffer with pains throughout their bodies. By the time that book was published, Morton was on his way to becoming the leading authority of the foot in the medical world.

If *The Human Foot* made Morton famous in the medical profession, it was his 1939 book, *Oh Doctor, My Feet!* written for the average person, that made him a household name.

After the release of *Oh Doctor, My Feet!,* there was no question that Dr. Dudley J. Morton was considered by both the public and the medical

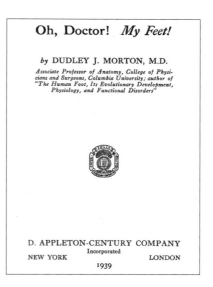

Oh, Doctor! *My Feet!*

by DUDLEY J. MORTON, M.D.

Associate Professor of Anatomy, College of Physicians and Surgeons, Columbia University; author of "The Human Foot, Its Evolutionary Development, Physiology, and Functional Disorders"

D. APPLETON-CENTURY COMPANY
Incorporated
NEW YORK   LONDON
1939

community as the leading authority on foot pain in this country. In that book, Morton explained to the average person why their feet really hurt, and what to do about it. Morton and the book were so celebrated that *Reader's Digest* asked him to write an article about the book, in their April 1939 issue. In the first paragraph of the *Reader's Digest* article, Morton wrote:

"Aching, pain galled feet are among the commonest afflictions besetting mankind. Seven of ten persons suffer from foot alignment of varying severity ranging from the nagging discomfort of corns to total disability from broken down feet."[8]

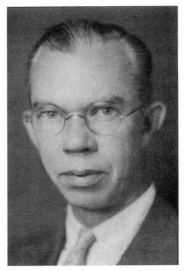

Dr. Morton in an undated photograph (Courtesy of Morton Family.)

Morton went on to say, in the *Reader's Digest* article, that then, as now, millions of dollars are spent annually on corrective shoes or other devices that are of questionable benefit in healing the foot. As always, he stated the two principal reasons for foot problems are the short first metatarsal bone and or the hypermobility of the first metatarsal bone. He continued to explain how to treat these conditions by putting a pad or a platform under the first metatarsal bone.

The book was also written about in the *New Yorker Magazine*[9] and was reviewed in dozens of newspapers across the country, from the *New York Times* to the *Oakland Tribune*. At about the same time, The American Medical Association also published an article for physicians that was written by Morton based on *Oh Doctor, My Feet!* Dudley J. Morton was one busy guy in 1939.

Throw Them Out!

In January 1942, Morton presented a paper at the Academy of Orthopedic Surgeons in Atlantic City. According to the *New York Times*, Morton made quite a sensation when he stated that 90% of arch supports that prop up thousands of feet ought to be thrown out the window. Furthermore, he said that the term "weak arches" should disappear from any discussion about the feet. Morton went on to say that other than high heels, shoes are not normally responsible for most foot problems. He also said that fallen arches are not the cause of most foot problems; the real problem is due to poorly distributed weight across the five metatarsal bones[10] (e.g., Morton's Toe). *Time* magazine, in their January 26, 1942 issue, also reported about Morton's presentation at this meeting.

From 1928 on, Morton was an associate professor of anatomy at the College of Physicians and Surgeons, Columbia University in New York. He not only taught and did research at Columbia, he also was on staff at Columbia Presbyterian Hospital, where he treated patients. He stayed at Columbia for sixteen years until he resigned on June 30, 1944.

Later Work

In December 1949, the *Reader's Digest* again published another article about Dr. Dudley J. Morton. This time it was a highly enthusiastic profile about him entitled "Something Wrong with Your Feet."[11] Paul de Kruif, who was a very famous author in his own right, wrote the piece. De Kruif was most noted for his book, *Microbe Hunters* that first published in 1926, and which is still in print today. De Kruif, who was a patient of Morton's, testified that arch supports failed him, while Morton's simple Toe Pad worked. He relates the story of how Morton discovered the importance of the short first metatarsal bone while looking at hundreds of X-rays, and how he developed the treatment for Morton's Toe. He then goes on to say how Morton received the scientific recognition he deserved, not only in the U.S. but overseas as well. De Kruif concluded *The Reader Digest* article by saying with admiration:

> "Thus thanks largely to Dr. Morton's pioneer work, one of the most common of foot defects need no longer cause widespread suffering."

Last Book

In 1952, with Dudley Dean Fuller, a Ph.D. in mechanical engineering (what is the story with these guys named Dudley!), Morton wrote his last book called *Human Locomotion and Body Form: A Study of Gravity and Man*.[12] It was well received and was republished overseas by an English publishing house.[13] There were of course,

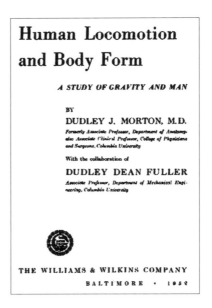

chapters on the short first metatarsal bone and hypermobility of the first metatarsal bone. But the book also reflected Dr. Morton's thirty-plus years of work on evolution that supported his belief that the only way humans could eventually stand erect and walk was because of inheritance over millions of years.

The Final Years

Morton's grandchildren Janice, Sandy and Chris (who are now in their fifties and sixties) have nothing but fond memories of their grandfather. At Thanksgiving, he insisted on carving the turkey at the family gathering. He regularly took his grandchildren to Ebbets Field, as he was

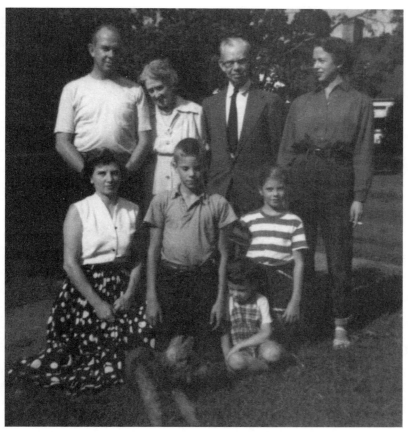

Dr. Morton and family, summer 1955. (Courtesy of Morton Family.)

an avid Brooklyn Dodgers fan. Right up to the end of his life, Morton was truly a "gentlemen's gentleman" even wearing a shirt and tie on summer outings.[14]

However, Morton, like many men of his time, was a chain smoker. His grandson, Chris, clearly recalls watching ball games on TV with his grandfather, as Dr. Morton lit one Kent cigarette after another. Unfortunately, it was this chain smoking that finally led to his death from cancer in May, 1960 at the age of seventy-six.[15]

In Chapter 14, I have provided more about the life and work of Dr. Dudley J. Morton that I hope you will find interesting."

Chapter 11

Janet Travell, MD

For years, on the wall of Janet Travell's office hung the following saying: "Life is like a bicycle, you don't fall off until you stop pedaling."[1] And pedal she did. I regret to inform you that Dr. Janet Travell only lived to be 95.

During her lifetime she not only helped develop a totally new understanding for why many of us hurt (Myofascial Pain Syndrome) and how to treat it; but she also served as the personal physician to two sitting Presidents of the United States and their families.

Like Dudley Morton, she understood how an abnormally working first metatarsal bone could cause foot pain. However, she took it further. She showed how a Morton's Toe could cause pain throughout the whole body by being a cause of *Myofascial Pain Syndrome.*

Dr. Travell was born in 1901 in New York City. She came from a family of physicians. Her father, Dr. Willard Travell, was recognized as an early pioneer in the treatment of pain. Janet's sister, Virginia, also became a doctor, and was a noted pediatrician.

Dr. Travell attended Wellesley College, where she graduated in 1922 with honors. She then went on to Cornell University Medical School where she earned her M.D. in 1926. During her four years in medical school,

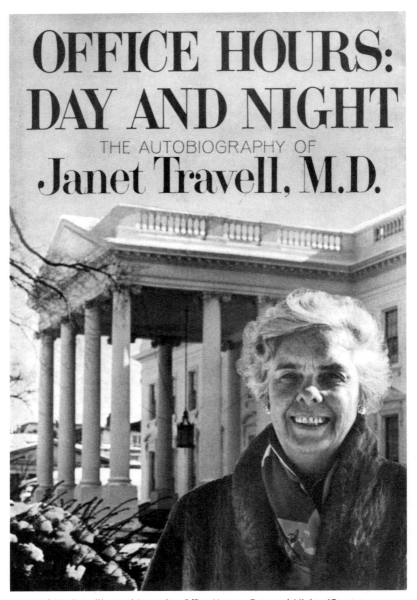

Cover of Dr. Travell's autobiography, Office Hours : Day and Night, (Courtesy Penguin Books USA)

she received the highest grades of any student.[2] This was clearly a sign of things to come.

After her postgraduate training in New York City, she accepted the position as a heart specialist at Sea View Hospital on Staten Island, a city hospital for tuberculosis in 1936. It would be at Sea View that Dr. Travell's life-long interest in muscle pain would begin. Most of her patients had very serious lung disease. But some of them complained more about the distressing pain in their shoulders and arms than about their lung illness. When she examined their shoulders and chest muscles, she discovered Myofascial trigger points for the first time.[3]

From this beginning at Sea View Hospital, her sixty-year-long study of Myofascial Pain Syndrome and trigger points therapy began to grow. In 1942, she published her first article about Myofascial Pain and Trigger Points in the *Journal of the American Medical Association*. It was coauthored with Dr. S. H. Rinzler and Dr. M. Herman.[4]

In 1952, she and Dr. Rinzler again coauthored another article called "The Myofascial Genesis of Pain." It appeared in *Postgraduate Medicine,* a prominent medical journal. It was a very important article in that it described for the first time trigger points in thirty-two muscles that caused Myofascial Pain Syndrome.[5]

By the 1950s, Janet Travell was already recognized as one of the leading experts in regard to the treatment of muscle pain and in general pain management.[6]

That is the reason she met her most famous patient.

John F. Kennedy

On May 26, 1955, Dr. Travell had her first appointment with her newly referred patient, Senator John F. Kennedy. It took place at her office at 9 West 16th Street in New York City.[7]

As she wrote in her autobiography, her recollections of that day were as follows, "At our first meeting, this thin young Senator on crutches could barely navigate the few steps down from the sidewalk into my ground floor office. Left-sided pain in his back and leg made it almost impossible for him to bear weight on that foot, and a stiff right knee since a football injury

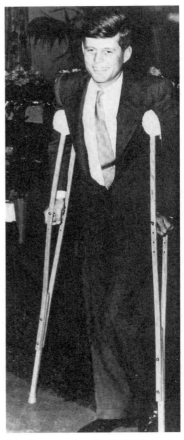

John F. Kennedy around 1952 (John F. Kennedy Library).

in his youth made it difficult for him to step up or down with his weight on the right leg, because that required bending of the right knee."[8]

She also stated that Kennedy required the assistance of his taxi driver just to help him down the few steps into her office. And, that he appeared pale, anemic and thin in spite of having a nice Florida suntan.[9]

To put it bluntly, John Fitzgerald Kennedy, United States Senator from the Commonwealth of Massachusetts, three days shy of his 38th birthday, was a total physical wreck.

His medical history was a nightmare. During his childhood, he would spend weeks on end in hospitals. In 1930, at the age of 13, he developed stomach problems. By 1934, he was diagnosed with colitis★ and was sent to the world famous Mayo Clinic for treatment.[10] In 1939, he had football injuries that would be the start of his life-long back problems. In 1943, as captain of the famous P.T. 109 during World War II, he received yet another major back injury when a Japanese destroyer sliced his ship in two.[11] The next year, he had a surgery to attempt to fix these back problems. It did not work.[12] In 1947, while on a trip to England, he was diagnosed with Addison's Disease.[13]★ In October 1954, seven months before his first visit with Dr. Travell, Kennedy had a fusion surgery done on his back. This was done yet again in an attempt to repair the earlier problems. It was a disaster. Shortly after the surgery, a complication arose. A serious infection occurred. Because of that, he was operated on again to remove the plates and three screws from the fusion surgery. Kennedy then went into a coma. He came so close to death that he was actually given the last rites of the Catholic Church.[14]

During a two-and-a-half-year period from 1955 to 1957, Kennedy was hospitalized a total of nine times for forty-five days. This included one 19-day stay and another two-week stay.[15]

John F. Kennedy was a mess.

Now, fast forward five-and-a-half years from that day in May 1955, when Kennedy met Travell for the first time. It is January 20, 1961, a very cold, snowy, and sunny day in Washington, D.C. (This writer remembers it clearly.) At exactly noon, John Fitzgerald Kennedy takes the oath of office to become the 35th President of the United States. The question is, how, within a relatively short period of time, did this "basket case" of a man, who couldn't even go down stairs without help, or walk without crutches, or even stand without severe pain, end up in the Oval Office? The answer is he got really lucky. Two important events happened at about the same time that changed his life. First, the drug cortisone became available to treat his Addison's disease, and then Janet Travell became his doctor.

Before the discovery of cortisone in the 1950s, the life expectancy of a person with Addisons disease was a lot shorter then that of the average person. Kennedy was very lucky to be in the right place at the right time. As Dr. Travell stated: "Senator Kennedy was the beneficiary of the discovery of adrenal hormones that was achieved by basic medical research. The timing of their clinical applications was right for him. He was a man of destiny."[16]

Well, we now know what cortisone did for John F. Kennedy but what did Dr. Janet Travell do?

The answer is simple. Because of her, John F. Kennedy was able to become the 35th President of the United States! It sounds unbelievable, but it is true.

Don't believe me. Below is an excerpt from a handwritten note that I obtained from the nice people at the John F. Kennedy Library in Boston. The note was dated June 23, 1961. It was written by Robert F. Kennedy to George McGovern regarding Dr. Travell's treatment of President Kennedy. It said:

"Dr. Travell has been working with him [JFK] for many years and if it was not for her, he would not presently be President of the United States."[17]

Please allow me to repeat that sentence:

"He would not presently be
President of the United States."

This remarkable statement by Robert F. Kennedy was referring to Dr. Travell's ongoing rehabilitation of President Kennedy's back problems. At the time he wrote this note, Robert F. Kennedy was the Attorney General of the United States and John F. Kennedy's brother and most trusted advisor. George McGovern was a good friend of the Kennedys who himself would be the Democratic candidate for President in 1972.

"She's a Genius"

That is how President Kennedy described Dr. Travell for "curing" the ailments that had troubled him for many years.[18]

From the first time they met in May 1955, until his death, Dr. Travell was always available to treat John F. Kennedy. Be it in Palm Beach Florida, Cape Cod, or in Washington, Travell was always there to treat him when needed. In January 1961, when President Kennedy moved into the White House, he appointed Dr. Travell to be the White House physician. She had the distinction of becoming the first female to be the personal physician to a President.[19] From her office in the basement of the White House, she continued to treat President Kennedy

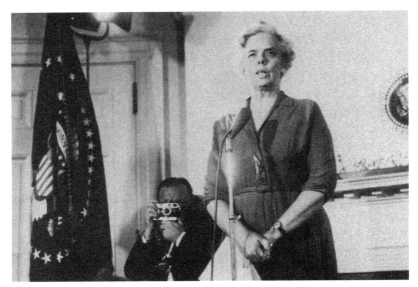

Dr. Travell at a White House press conference in 1961 (John F. Kennedy Library).

on a regular basis. She most often gave him Novocaine injections in his back to treat the muscle spasms causing his Myofascial pain. Besides injections, Travell also prescribed physical therapy when needed. In the *New York Times* of June 14, 1961, the headline read "Super-sonic Rays Used on Kennedy." The story went on to relate how JFK was prescribed ultrasound therapy by Dr. Travell for low back strain.[20]

The Rocking Chair

For those of you who were not around at the time John F. Kennedy was President, he was famous for being seen in his rocking chair. He was always photographed or filmed sitting in it. Be it in a news reel, at a meeting with a world leader, or in a still photograph where he was just

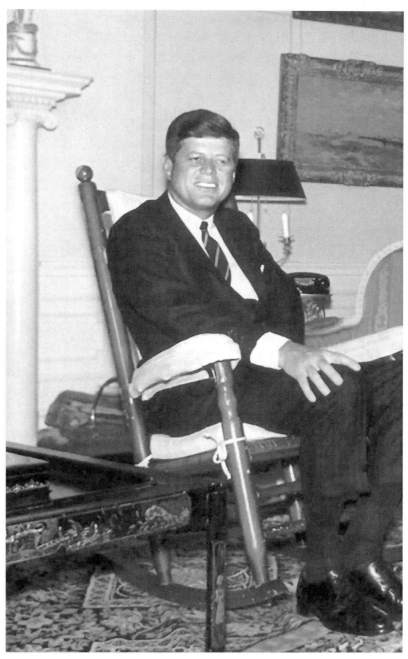

President Kennedy on March 19, 1962 sitting in the North Carolina porch rocking chair prescribed for him by Dr. Travell (John F. Kennedy Library).

147

thinking, there were hundreds of images of John F. Kennedy sitting in his cane rocking chair.

It was Dr. Travell who introduced Kennedy to the benefits of the rocking chair. She used rocking chairs as a treatment for back pain for many years, even before she met John F. Kennedy. She felt it decreased lower back strain by keeping the muscles moving, and often prescribed it to her patients. At his very first appointment with Dr. Travell, in her office in May 1955, Kennedy sat in an "old style North Carolina porch rocking chair with woven cane seat and back."[21] It was "love at first sit." He commented that sitting on it did make him feel better. Immediately following that first visit, Kennedy left Travell's office and went directly to New York Hospital where he was admitted and stayed for a week under her care. The first thing Dr. Travell did for her patient, after he was admitted into the hospital, was to personally take the rocking chair from her office and bring it to Kennedy's hospital room for him to use.[22] From that day forward, JFK always had rocking chairs nearby. That is how it all started. Throughout his White House years, Kennedy's oak rocker with the cane seat with the Presidential Seal on the back, became one of the emblems of his Presidency. It was Travell who made this lasting contribution to presidential folklore with the popularity of the rocking chair.[23]

LBJ and Later Years

After President Kennedy died, President Lyndon B. Johnson asked Dr. Travell to stay on as the White House physician and she agreed. For the next year-and-a-half, she treated not only President Johnson, but the entire first family. In 1965, she resigned as the White House physician so she could continue her life's work of writing and teaching about Myofascial pain, which she did for the next thirty years. For the vast majority of this time, she was also on staff at George Washington University Medical School, where she ended her career with the highest honor which one could receive: the title "Professor Emeritus of Medicine." All of her medical papers are also kept at the Gellman Library at George Washington University in Washington D.C. Dr. Travell's autobiography was published in 1968. It was called *Office Hours: Day and Night*.[24] It is a fascinating book that gives you a front row seat not only to Travell's life and times, but also a grand view of the twentieth century. In 1984, the first volume of *Myofascial Pain & Dysfunction: The Trigger Point Manual* was published with the second volume being published in 1990.[25] These two books are the "gold standard" for Myofascial pain and its treatments.

Dr. Janet Travell died on August 1, 1997 at the age of 95. Because of her lifelong work, she left the world a much better place than the one she came into almost a century before. Thousands of people, are better, and will be better because of her almost seventy year remarkable career.

Part 2

Chapter 12

More About Myofascial Pain and Morton's Toe

In Chapter 7, I wrote about Myofascial Pain Syndrome, its relationship with Morton's Toe, and how you can hurt all over from it. In this chapter, I will tell you more about this relationship.

How a Morton's Toe Can Make Your Teeth Hurt

While I was writing this book, one of my long time patients came in to see me. He was a retired dentist who earlier in his life did some research on *Temporomandibular Joint Pain* (TMJ). This is a painful muscular condition affecting the jaw which in turn can also effect the teeth, neck, eyes and ears and even cause headaches. I mentioned the work I was doing regarding Dr. Travell and Myofascial Pain Syndrome, and we both wondered if in fact the Morton's Toe could be causing TMJ. We both laughed when I said, "Wouldn't it be something if the day comes when you went to a doctor for treatment of Temporomandibular Joint Pain, and he told you to take your shoes and socks off so he can put a pad on your feet to treat your painful jaw and teeth?"

Well, guess what? That's exactly what Travell and Simmons said. In spite of my studying their books for many years, I somehow missed what they had to say about Temporomandibular Joint Pain and the "Dudley J. Morton's Foot" (Morton's Toe).

In Volume 1 of their book, Travell and Simons stated:

> "Surprisingly in the lower extremity muscles can interact with tense muscles of the head and neck to restrict movement of the latter. Release of tension in the lower extremity muscles by inactivation of their TP's (trigger points) such as those perpetuated by a **short first, long second metatarsal relationship** (emphasis added) may at once increase a TP restricted interincisal opening of the jaws by 20 or 30%"[1]

They went on to say it is remarkable that Trigger Points activity in the leg muscles due to the Dudley J. Morton Foot and other muscles can restrict the mouth from opening.[2] In addition, once these Trigger Points are inactivated the jaw muscles can relax, with the end result that there is a marked increase in opening at once. Along the way, your teeth can stop hurting because the muscle spasms causing your pain are gone. This is assuming you treat the underlying Morton's Toe that is the cause of the problem to start with.

These restrictions of the jaw muscles can also cause pains of the cheek, eyes, eyebrows, ears, and be the cause of headaches. So, the aim is to stop the Morton's Toe from activating the trigger points.[3]

Wow! So a Morton's Toe can make your teeth hurt and cause a lot of other problems. What are you waiting for? Put the Toe Pad on your foot if you haven't already!

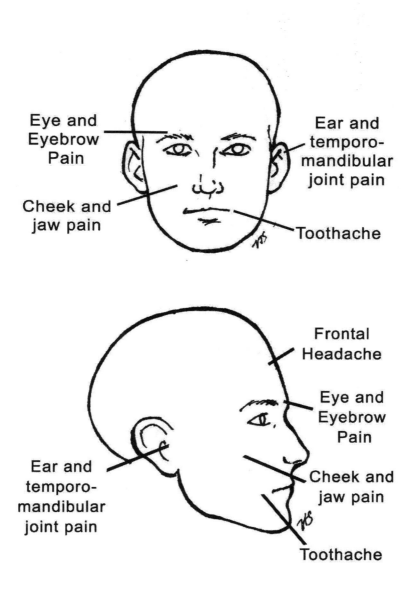

Eye and Eyebrow Pain

Ear and temporo-mandibular joint pain

Cheek and jaw pain

Toothache

Frontal Headache

Eye and Eyebrow Pain

Ear and temporo-mandibular joint pain

Cheek and jaw pain

Toothache

The above diagrams show places on the head where you can have Myofascial trigger points because of a Morton's Toe.

More About Myofascial Pain and Fibromyalgia

In June 2007, I was very fortunate to have a phone conversation with Dr. David Simmons, co-author with Dr. Travell of Myofascial Pain and Dysfunction: The Trigger Point Manual. During that conversation, I asked Dr. Simmons about the relationship between Fibromyalgia and Myofascial Pain Syndrome. He said that he felt that some patients with fibromyalgia might also have Myofascial trigger points that could be making their fibromyalgia worse. And there are people being treated for fibromyalgia when in fact what they really have is Myofascial Pain that needs to be treated.[4]

True, these two conditions are very much alike, but they are also different. They differ in that, according to The American College of Rheumatology, you must have pain in at least eleven of eighteen specified tender points for at least three months to be diagnosed with Fibromyalgia.[5] But in Myofascial Pain Syndrome, the pain is regional and accompanied by trigger points.[6] It is important to find out which one you have. But it is also important to determine if you have a Morton's Toe because it could be the real cause of either of these painful conditions. As before, be very careful in using the Toe Pad in the beginning if you have a serious case of fibromyalgia. The Toe Pad is serious medicine, and with any type of medicine, it can have side effects. Go slow!

Treatments

There are several well-established treatments for Myofascial pain. The basic aim of these treatments is to "inactivate" the trigger points in the muscles that are causing your pain. The two most popular are Stretch and Spray, and Trigger Point injections

I. Stretch and Spray

Stretch and Spray is the workhouse of Myofascial therapy. In the 1940s Dr. Travell became aware that freezing sprays could be used as a way to relieve Myofascial Pain by distracting the painful trigger points of the muscle.[7] Since then these sprays have been one of the most popular treatments for Myofascial Pain. Once the trigger point is calmed down with the freezing spray, it can be stretched, allowing deactivation of it to take place. Patient's referred pain is also reduced by stretch and spray.[8]

You can see a very good video of the stretch and spray technique at http://video.aol.com/video-detail/stretching-y-spray-and-stretch-peroneos/3294540709. The audio on the tape is in Spanish but it is still easy to understand.

II. Trigger Point Injections

Some muscles just don't respond to Stretch and Spray. When this occurs Trigger point injections are an alternative. They normally contain a local anesthetic. This is performed in the doctor's office and not in a hospital. Several trigger points can be injected in one visit.

One injection can relieve pain in the muscle from minutes to months depending on the severity of the trigger point.[9] The one major advantage with an injection is that after the area is numb a much more comprehensive stretching of the muscle is possible to deactivate the Trigger Points in question. These injections have been shown to reduce pain, increase circulation to the muscle and increase range of motion.

Morton's Toe has been shown to be a cause of Myofascial Pain Syndrome, and most probably Fibromyalgia. With each passing year, Myofascial Pain has been more and more acknowledged as the real underlying reason for many of our chronic discomforts. The good news is that because of the work of Dr. Dudley J. Morton and Dr. Janet Travell, millions of people with Myofascial Pain may now feel better.

Chapter 13

Diabetic Ulcers, Amputations and The Morton's Toe

Based on the most current U.S. government information available, about 82,000 diabetics had amputations
in 2002.[1] I am very depressed by those numbers
because as a long time professional member of the
American Diabetes Association and a Certified Wound
Specialist,[2] I know that some of those amputations could
have been avoided if the patient and or their doctors only
knew more about Dr. Morton's Toe.

In order for an amputation to occur the patient first
must develop a wound (ulcer).

Diabetic Foot Ulcers

Foot ulcers first start out as being sores or calluses on the
skin. They are caused by some type of irritation. With
time, these sores or calluses can break down, causing a
wound or opening in your foot to occur. This wound or
opening is an ulcer. Once this happens, the foot can get
infected, eventually leading to gangrene★ and possible
amputation. But in order for the skin to start breaking
down, certain complications must be present. Two of these
complications are poor circulation and nerve damage.
Many diabetics have poor circulation and nerve damage,
but most of them do not get foot ulcers.

Why?

Those diabetics who do get foot ulcers also have one other complication. This is abnormal stress, strains and other trauma going through their feet like we see in patients with Morton's Toe or other types of foot problems. The combination of poor circulation, nerve damage, and trauma (from Morton's Toe) is called the Diabetic Foot Triad (Fig. 13-1). This is a trifecta you really do not want to have. The three of them together, if left untreated in a diabetic, can lead to the formation of a foot ulcer or worse.

Please allow me to repeat this again, because it is incredibly important. There are millions of diabetics walking around with ice-cold, numb feet who don't have foot ulcers. The reason they do not get ulcers despite their severe diabetic condition is because their feet work fairly normally. Because of this, they do not have any unusual stress or trauma going through their foot, which

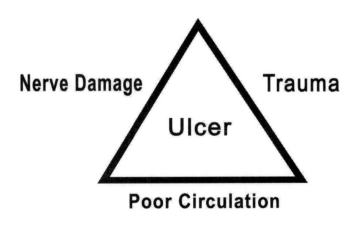

THE DIABETIC FOOT TRIAD

Fig. 13-1 Foot triad diagram.

can cause the feet to break down. A Morton's Toe or other foot problems can cause this trauma. That is why some people get diabetic ulcers and some don't. Like with non-diabetics, your foot health depends a great deal upon the feet you got from Mom or Dad.

One warning: if you have very poor circulation to your feet, you are always prone to get infections, regardless of any foot problem being present.

From Ulcer to Amputation

If an ulcer does not heal, it can end up causing an amputation of the foot. One of the major reasons for this worsening condition is due to the ongoing trauma to the feet that caused the ulcer to form in the first place. If this happens, the ulcer can stay open, then get infected, which then can lead to an amputation. In order to stop this ongoing daily trauma, the patient with a diabetic ulcer must be treated with a Toe Pad or an orthotic. When this is combined with one of our new wound healing treatments, the patient can have a better chance of healing and avoiding an amputation.

The best part of my job is getting to meet and treat some really neat people. One of these patients was Bill Allred. He was a drummer, but not your average one. He toured for about two years as the drummer for Country and Western superstar Kenny Chesney. Bill is and was an insulin diabetic. From the constant banging of the drum's foot pedal, Bill got an irritation, than an ulcer, then a serious infection of his left foot. This problem forced him to quit Kenny Chesney's band and give up drumming. His condition did not improve.

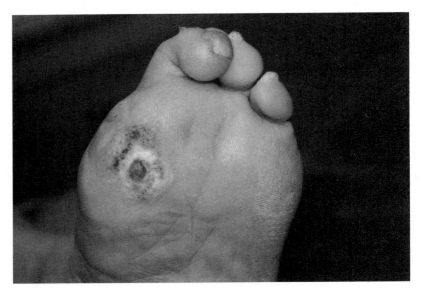

Diabetic ulcer with an amputation.

By the time he came to my office, he'd already had numerous foot surgeries to save his foot. His left big toe was already amputated and he had a very large ulcer under the first metatarsal head of the left foot that was wide open and very painful.

He said several doctors already had healed the ulcer numerous times, but it continued to keep breaking down, reopening, and causing him great pain and distress. Bill was sick and tired of the constant draining of the wound and hoped I would be able to do something about it. After treating him for several months, I was able to get the ulcer healed. The question was would it stay healed. I knew he had a Morton's Toe so I made him an orthotic that treated the abnormal ongoing daily trauma caused by his Morton's Toe, the real cause of his ulcer never totally healing. Bill was really happy. He felt so good that he was able to go back to drumming. This worked fine for several months until one night he overdid it while playing at a "Toga Party" (no kidding) and his ulcer started to open up again. Luckily, he came in right away and I was able to treat this new wound without any great damage being done. I did have to send his orthotic back to the laboratory to be fitted with the "toga party protection package" (a thicker Toe Pad!)

The Diabetic Shoe Program

If you already have a diabetic shoe from Medicare, you are very lucky. The reason is that the molded insole that came in your shoe (you should have received three pairs) can be removed, and you can easily attach a Toe Pad to the top or bottom of it. If your foot and/or body does not feel better after wearing the Toe Pad for awhile just remove it from the diabetic insole.

If you are a diabetic and you have corns, calluses, or heel pain, do not wait, see a podiatrist at once. As a diabetic, you must be proactive. What this means is that you cannot wait for an ulcer to appear on your foot; you should not give it a chance to happen. You do not have the luxury like everyone else of fixing a problem when it appears. As a diabetic, you must prevent it before it starts! Any wound care specialist will tell you it is a thousand times easier to prevent an ulcer from appearing than trying to heal one. By being proactive you will not become one of those 80,000 or so amputations this year, many due to a Morton's Toe.

Chapter 14

More About Dudley Joy Morton, M.D.

In Chapter 10, I wrote about the life of Dr. Dudley Morton. Here is more of his story.

1922

If there was one year that launched Dudley J. Morton, M.D. into the public arena, and started to establish him as a medical expert, it was 1922. His first taste of notoriety came on April 16, 1922 when the *New York Times* ran a story about one "John Daniels." John Daniels, you see, was a young gorilla that had been turned over to the American Museum of Natural History for dissection after his death.[1] Morton got the job of working on John Daniels and writing about him. Later in 1922, he gained more notoriety when he published two more papers on the evolution of the human foot.

The Real Hannibal Lecter Meets Dr. Dudley Morton

Albert H. Fish was one of the most infamous killers of the first half of the twenty century. Fish was a grandfatherly man who specialized in murdering and cannibalizing children. He claimed to have molested 100 children. He was known as America's first serial killer. You will find an article about him in Wikipedia. There are no less than two dozen web sites about and or including him. A movie was made about his life in 2006. (Albertfishfilm. com) Finally, for all you movie fans, Albert Fish was the model for Hannibal Lecter, the monster in the "Silence of the Lambs" films.

So, what does this guy have to do with Dudley Morton? In an interesting but gruesome aside, and as a testament to Morton's expertise in anatomy, he was called upon to testify for the State of New York against Fish in a murder trial. Please let the March 16, 1935, *Albuquerque Journal* explain.

> WHITE PLAINS, N.Y. March 15. The state rested its case against Albert H. Fish for the slaying of 10 year old Grace Budd in Supreme Court today after it had called to the stand a Columbia University anatomist to reconstruct, with human bones, the skeleton of a little decapitated girl.[2]

(Sorry about that). The article stated that Dr. Dudley J. Morton, of the College of Physicians and Surgeons, testified that based on the bones from the child's body, he found that she was between 10 and 12 years old and was between 51-52 inches tall. The State of New York saved Dr. Morton for their last and most important witness and then they rested their case. Thanks to Dudley Morton, Albert H. Fish was convicted as one of the worst serial killers of the 20th century. Fish was finally executed for the murder of Grace Budd in the electric chair on January 16, 1936 in New York State's Sing Sing prison. Nice going Dudley!

More on OH, DOCTOR! MY FEET!

Besides the article in *Readers Digest* (page 134) "Oh, Doctor! My Feet!" was reviewed and written about in many newspapers and magazines across the country.

On February 26, 1939, the *New York Times*[3] reviewed the book and said "Dr. Morton does use a narrative presentation, which makes it easy to understand. But does not try to be popular as he tells the readers about the true facts about their foot troubles."

In the May 13, 1939, *New Yorker* Magazine, celebrated American humorist S.J. Pearlman wrote a story called, *Boy Meets Girl Meets Foot*.[4] In it, he gives a very funny review of *Oh, Doctor! My Feet!* and makes some fun of Dr. Morton. But over all it was a very nice article about the book, by a very noted and highly respected writer (Pearlman), in one of the most important magazines of its time. In fact, sixty years later, in the year 2000, "Boy Meets Girl Meets Foot" was considered one of Pearlman's finest pieces of writing when it was included in the book *Most of the Most of S.J. Pearlman*[5], a collection of Pearlman's best works.

Previously in Chapter 10, I wrote about a meeting in early 1942 at which Dr. Morton spoke before the Academy of Orthopedic Surgeons in Atlantic City, N.J. What he said must have been important because both Time Magazine and the *New York Times* reported about it.

The *Time Magazine* article appeared in the January 26, 1942 issue and was titled "Mirrored Feet." The article told how Morton used an invention called a barograph. The data collected by Morton from the barography was then used to diagnose the patient's foot problems.

Morton was so impressed with this device that he said he was sure that the barograph will be as useful to orthopedists as the cardiograph is to heart specialists.[6]

The previous week, the January 18, 1942's New York Times' "Science In the News" section also wrote a long article about Dr. Morton, the Atlantic City meeting, and the barography.[7] They said the same thing that Time Magazine would write the following week, except they enclosed in the article a really nice picture of someone standing on the barography. The caption on the picture read *"Finding Out Why Feet Ache."*

As I also wrote in Chapter 10, Dr. Morton's last major work was *Human Locomotion and Body Form,* published by Williams and Williams in 1952.[8] In 1953, the book was published in England by Bailliere, Tindall, and Cox Ltd.

To the best of my knowledge, the following is the first complete list of the books and articles writen by and about Dudley J. Morton, M.D.

Books written by Dr. Morton:
- *The Grampa's Toy Shop.* 1922, Grampa Co.
- *Human Anatomy: double dissection method,* 1934 New York, Columbia University Press.
- *The Human Foot, its evolution, physiology and functional disorder.* 1935 New York Columbia University Press. Reprinted 1964 Hafner Publishing Co.
- *Oh, Doctor! My Feet!* 1939 Appleton-Century Company, Incorporated, New York and London.
- *Manual of Human Cross Section Anatomy,* 1944 Baltimore, The Williams & Wilkins Company.
- *Human Locomotion and Body Form; a Study of Gravity and Man,* 1952 (with Dudley Dean Fuller) Baltimore, The Williams & Wilkins Company, Published overseas by Bailliere, Tindall, and Cox Ltd., 1952, London.

Articles written by Dr. Morton:

- Mans' Descent: Clears Points in Lecture on Evolution of Human Foot, April 21, 1922, *The New York Times.*
- Evolution of The Human Foot (1922) Am. *Journal of Physical Anthropology*, vol. V, no. 4 October-December.
- Evolution of the Longitudional Arch of The Human Foot (1924) *J. Bone & Joint Surgery* 6: 56-90.
- Mechanism of the Normal Foot and of Flat Foot: Part 1. (1924) *J. Bone Joint Surg.* Am. 6: 368-386.
- The Peroneus Tertius Muscle in Gorillas, (1924) *Anatomical Record,* Vol. 27, no. 5.
- Signifant Characteristics of The Neanderthal Foot, (1926) *Natural History,* Vol. XXVI no. 3, pp. 310-314.
- The Relation of Evolution to Medicine, (1926) *Science* Oct 22; 64 (1660) pp. 394-396.
- Human Origin. Correlation of Previous Studies of Primate Feet and Poster with Other Morphologic Evidence, (1927) *Am.* Journal of Physical Anthropology, Vol. X no. 2.
- Metatarsus Atavicus: The Identification of a Distinctive Type of Foot Disorder, (1927) *J. Bone Joint Surg.* Am., 9: 531-544.
- Hypermobility of the First Metatarsal Bone: The Interlinking Factor Between Metatarsalgia and Longitudinal Arch Strains, (1928) *J. Bone Joint Surg.* Am., 10: 187-196.
- Structural Factors in Static Disorders of The Human Foot, (1930) *Am J Surgery* 9: 315-326.
- Notes of Foot Disorders Among Natives of the Belgian Congo, (1931) *J. Bone Joint Surg.* Am., 13: 311-318.
- (Co authored with Earl T. Engle) The Angle of Gait: A Study Based Upon Exhamination of the Feet of Central African Natives, (1932) *J. Bone Joint Surg.* Am., 14: 741-754.
- Physiological Considerations in the Treatment of Foot Deformities, (1937) *J. Bone Joint Surg.* Am., 19: 1052-1056.
- Oh Doctor, My Feet!, *The Readers Digest,* April 1939 95-98.

Newspapers and Magazines Articles, written about, citing or quoting Dr. Dudley J. Morton (*The New York Times* wrote about him man times over almost forty years. Here are some of those articles.)

- April 16, 1922, JOHN DANIELS TOE WITNESS FOR DARWIN: Shape Of It Help To Prove Man Could Have Descendent From A Gorilla.
- April 2, 1926, SEMI-ERECT STAGE OF MAN DENIED; Dr. D.J. Morton Tells Anatomists In New Haven Session Development Was Distinct.
- September 8, 1926, LINKS EVOLUTION WITH MEDICAL LORE; Dr. Morton Tells British Physicians Visiting Yale Doctors Must Carry On Its Study.
- March 2, 1931, BRINGS FIVE GORILLAS FOR APE STUDY HERE.
- November 5, 1935, WOMEN ADVISED TO LIMIT WEARING HIGH HEEL SHOES TO THE EVENING.
- November 10, 1935, SIDELIGHTS OF THE WEEK: LADIES AND HEELS, If Women Wore Tall Heels only in the Evenings, They Would Suffer Much Less From Foot Disorders.
- November 29, 1939, CARE FOR DISCONTENTED FEET: Book Review of OH, DOCTOR! MY FEET! BY DUDLEY J. MORTON M.D.
- January 18, 1942, SCIENCE IN THE NEWS, Finding Out Why Feet Ache.
- September 7, 1952, SCIENCE IN REVIEW; Biomechanics Throw New Light on Evolution of Man As A Result Of Locomotion and Gravity.

And finally the *New York Times* wrote on:
- May 23, 1960, DUDLEY MORTON, SURGEON, 76, DIES.

Other newspapers and publications that wrote about Dudley J. Morton, M.D.

THE 1920s:
- *The Bee,* Danville, Virginia, April 25, 1922.
- *The Bridgeport Telegram,* Bridgeport Connecticut, May 4, 1922.
- *The Gettysburg Times,* Gettysburg, Pennsylvania, April 16, 1924.
- *The Star and Sentinel,* Gettysburg, Pennsylvania, April 19, 1924.
- *The Bridgeport Telegram,* Bridgeport Connecticut, December 12, 1924.
- *San Mateo Times,* San Mateo, California, May 20, 1926.
- *The Port Arthur News,* Port Arthur Texas, September 30, 1926.
- *Olean Evening Times,* Olean, New York October 2, 1926.
- *Decatur Herald,* Decatur, Illinois, January 16, 1928.

THE 1930s:
- *The Lowell Sun,* Lowell Massachusetts, October 31, 1931.
- *The Syracuse Herald,* Syracuse, New York, October 28, 1932.
- *Wisconsin Daily Tribune,* Wisconsin Rapids Wisconsin October 29, 1932.
- *The Helena Independent,* Helena, Montana November 1, 1932.
- *Modesto News-Herald,* Modesto, California, November 3, 1932.
- *The News, Frederick,* Maryland November 7, 1932.
- *The Frederick Post,* Frederick Maryland, November 8, 1932.
- *Ironwood Daily Globe,* Ironwood, Michigan, November 10, 1932.
- *Reno Evening Gazette,* Reno Nevada, November 10, 1932.
- *The Lima News,* Lima Ohio, July 23, 1933.
- *Fitchburg Sentinel,* Fitchburg Massachusetts, March 15, 1935.

- *Albuquerque Journal,* Albuquerque New Mexico, March 16, 1935.
- *The Kingston Daily,* Freeman Kingston, New York March 15, 1935.
- *Dunkirk Observer,* Dunkirk, New York, February 15, 1938.
- *Indiana Weekly,* Indiana, Pennsylvania, April 14, 1938.
- *Fredericksburg News,* Fredericksburg, Iowa April 14, 1938
- *The Daily Courier,* Connellsville, Pennsylvania, February 10, 1939.
- *Oakland Tribune,* Oakland California, March 7, 1939.
- *The Circleville Herald,* Circleville, Ohio, March 18, 1939.
- *Florence Morning News,* Florence, South Carolina, March 24, 1939.
- *Middletown Times Herald,* Middletown, New York, March 25, 1939.
- *Appleton Post-Crescent,* Appleton Wisconsin May 27, 1939.
- *The Circleville Herald,* Circleville, Ohio, July 14, 1939.
- *The Time Recorder,* Zanesville, Ohio, July 21, 1939.
- *Middletown Times Herald,* Middletown, New York, July 21, 1939.
- *The Hammond Times,* Hammond Indiana, July 21, 1939.
- *The Daily Courier,* Connellsville, Pennsylvania, July 21, 1939.
- *The Vidette-Messenger,* Valparaiso, Indiana, July 26, 1939.
- *The Daily Courier,* Connellsville, Pennsylvania, October 2, 1939.
- *Coshocton Tribune,* Coshocton, Ohio, November 7, 1939.
- *The New Yorker Magazine,* "Boy Meets Girl Meets Foot", S.J. Perleman, May 1939.

THE 1940s:
- *Time Magazine,* Mirrored Feet, January 26, 1942.
- *The Lethbridge Herald,* Lethbridge, Alberta, October 12, 1943.
- *Kingsport News,* Kingsport Tennessee, October 12, 1943.
- *The Cullman Democrat,* Cullman Alabama, May 25, 1944.
- *Modesto Bee News-Herald,* Modesto, California, January 7, 1946.

- *The Fresno Bee Republican,* Fresno California, January 7, 1946.
- *Gazette and Bulletin,* Williamsport Pennsylvania, March 22, 1947.
- *Waterloo Daily Courier,* Waterloo Iowa, December 5, 1947.
- *The Marion Star,* Marion Ohio, December 11, 1947.
- *The Vidette-Messenger,* Valparaiso, Indiana, December 12, 1947.
- *The Reader's Digest,* "Something Wrong with Your Feet", Paul de Kruif, December 1949.

THE 1950s:
- *Pasadena Independent,* Pasadena California, May 19, 1959.
- *Nevada State Journal,* Reno Nevada, October 8, 1959.
- *The Post Standard,* Syracuse New York, October 23, 1959.

Chapter 15

Arch Supports and the Scam that Goes With Them

For years, the public has had the idea that if their feet hurt, the simplest thing to do to take care of them was to get a pair of arch supports or insoles. This is a myth. I hope that after reading this book, you now understand that contrary to everything you have ever been told, "supporting your arch" is not the answer, or even the proper treatment for most real foot problems. Sure, arch supports can make you feel better by cushioning the arch. However, they do not take care of any of the basic problems of the muscles, ligaments, bones or tendons of the foot which are the real reasons for most of our foot and body pains. Every year, millions of people buy arch supports only to find out that their foot problems do not get any better, and they have wasted their time and money. If this was not bad enough, most foot doctors (including myself) have seen numerous patients with foot problems that have been made worse by these inferior arch supports.

Moreover, a Morton's Toe Pad or a Shoe Insert at 1% of the cost can treat most foot problems as well—if not better—than any of those overpriced arch supports or insoles.

Dr. Morton on Arch Supports

As far back as sixty-five years ago, Dr. Dudley Morton

knew that arch supports were of doubtful use in treating foot problems.

As I wrote in Chapter 10, in January 1942, Morton presented a paper at the Academy of Orthopedic Surgeons in Atlantic City, where he stated that 90% of the arch supports that prop up thousands of feet ought to be thrown out the window. He also said that fallen arches are not the cause of most foot problems, but rather the real problem is due to poorly distributed weight across the five metatarsal bones (Morton's Toe). He also noted that the real reason for most foot problems, including fallen arches, is due to problems of the first metatarsal bone.

Fraudulent Claims

> "You can fool some of the people all of the time, and all of the people some of the time, but you cannot fool all of the people all of the time."—Abraham Lincoln

There are big big bucks to be made in selling pre-made arch supports and insoles. It is an industry that makes hundreds of millions of dollars a year. They are sold everywhere from special chain stores that sell nothing but arch supports and insoles to a guy selling them out of the trunk of his car. The one common denominator is that these "things" are sold based on false hopes and fraudulent claims. The people selling them have as much knowledge and training about the human foot and why you really hurt as the nice person who asked you if you want paper or plastic at the grocery checkout counter. The one thing they have been trained to do is repeat the script they were taught to sell these "things" to the hurting public. The truth is that if you are hurting, it does not take much to convince you to buy something that you hope will give you relief. The worst part of this story is that once you buy these arch supports or insoles, you are stuck with them regardless of whether you paid ten bucks or hundreds of dollars. However, the public and state authorities are catching on, as you will see shortly.

During the summer, there is a monthly street fair in my home town of Panama City, FL. Thousands of people attend. It is a very popular event with music, food, old cars and vendors selling all types of merchandise. The last time I went, there was a booth selling something called "massaging insoles" for $39.99. Hanging in the booth was a large banner saying that these insoles provided relief from heel spurs, low back pain, burning feet, fibromyalgia, Morton's neuroma, plantar fasciitis, bunions, calluses, and varicose veins. The only thing it did not claim to treat was "E.D." These claims are absolutely ridiculous and outrageous and are not based on anything substantial. I examined the insoles and found there was nothing therapeutic about them. In fact, this same insole or something very similar, can be bought for about four dollars through a catalogue or online. Go to a discount store and you can buy them for about six to eight dollars.

The Arch Support Chain Stores or There is No Magic Arch Support

The biggest change in the way arch supports and insoles are marketed is with the recent invention of stores that sell nothing but them. Not that long ago, you could go into any drug store and buy a pair of arch supports or insoles for about three to five dollars. But that was before someone came up with the lucrative idea of reinventing and repackaging arch supports and charging hundreds of dollars for them. Because of that, we now have franchised chain stores across the country that specialize in selling pre-made, off-the-shelf arch support or insoles. There is nothing special about these arch supports; there is nothing magical about these arch supports except for the way the buyer is being uniquely ripped off. You see, the same arch supports or insoles sold in these chain stores for $200 to $400 can be bought by anyone for about ten to twenty dollars at pharmacies, discount stores, or through catalogues. If you go online, Dr Scholl's™ is selling the same thing or a similar arch support for about nine dollars. You can even buy them from the T.V. for $19.95 (plus shipping and handling). The only difference is that in the chain store they put on a "Dog and Pony Show★" to convince the buyer that they need these overpriced insoles. This Dog and Pony Show consists of having the customer walk on a mat that makes an imprint of their foot. It looks impressive to the customer but in reality, it means nothing. They then tell the customer (sorry, you are not a "patient") that their arch has fallen and they need an arch support. Again, this is garbage only being said to con you into buying one of the stores' overpriced products.

The chain store arch supports are mostly made overseas. They are all mass-produced, based on standard shoe sizes (not on your foot). The wholesale cost to the chain store is about three to five dollars per pair and then it is marked up about 100 times! It has to be considered one of the greatest mass-marketing ploys of recent times. Imagine taking a three-dollar item and selling it for $300! This is America, and if you want to pay $300 to $400 for a hard plastic or rubber arch support from China that certainly is your right. The major problem arises when the arch supports or insoles do not work as advertised and the customer wants a cash refund from the chain store, but they are totally refused one. I will tell you more about this swindle shortly, but first I must tell you about the background of the salespeople selling you these over-priced insoles and arch supports.

Sales People

The sales people who sell arch supports and insoles in the chain store have no medical background. They **cannot** explain to you why your feet really hurt because they have no clue why they hurt. In addition, it is illegal for them to do so.

The sales people **cannot** determine for you if any of your problems were or were not due to a serious systemic disease such as diabetes, arthritis, bursitis, poor circulation, nerve damage, back problems, or gout.

The sales people **cannot** tell you if your pains in your arch or foot are caused by a bone that is broken, an abnormal bone growth, or a bone tumor.

When you buy arch supports from these stores, you have no idea of the background of the sales person with whom you are dealing. For or all you know, they could have been selling mobile homes before this job. Did I say "mobile homes?"

Yep, Another True Story

Throughout this book, I have told you many true stories. In many ways, the following story is the most important one. In this part of the United States, mobile homes are a very popular form of housing. Several years ago, I went with a friend who was shopping for a doublewide mobile home. A young salesman showed us the different models. We started to talk and eventually the young salesperson admitted to me that he was starting a new job the following week. When I asked him about it, he said that he was going to work for a national chain of stores that sold nothing but arch supports. He indicated that his friend worked in the Tallahassee, Florida store and was making a "killing" from the commissions on these things. I asked him if he had any experience in selling arch supports or any medical background. He said no, but that the company would teach him what to say and how to sell them. I did not voluntarily tell him that I spent the last 25 years looking at feet everyday.

The Choice is Yours

The salespeople in the arch support stores are not there to help you. They are there to help themselves, by making their commissions. The point is that for the same hundreds of dollars you would be spending on a pre made arch support you could be seeing a doctor who would really determine the reasons for your painful feet. So the choice is yours. You could either go see a podiatrist who has years of experience in treating the foot, or a man or woman who has years of experience in sales. Finally, there is another bonus in getting the proper care. Insurance companies would never pay for the arch support from the chain store, while (depending on your policy) they should pay for you to see your local podiatrist to find out why you are really hurting, and then pay for the proper treatment. Like I said above, do not assume you need an arch support just because your feet hurt. You need to find out the answer for certain.

I will now document the scam/rip-off going on across the country when most of these chain stores make fraudulent misrepresentations about their products and then absolutely refuse to give any refund when these overpriced arch supports don't work.

The National Ripoff

Television stations across the country have ran numerous reports about complaints made by consumers concerning alleged fraudulent sales practices of these franchised arch support stores, and their refusals to give ANY refunds to unhappy customers. Here are only some of them:

WISC-TV in Madison, Wisconsin ran an on-air piece called "Not So Good 'Good Feet'". It reported that state consumer protection officials are sending 41 complaints against the *Good Feet Store* to the Justice Department for investigation after allegations that the store's infomercials are fraudulent representations of their products. Some consumers complained that after spending hundreds of dollars on arch supports that did not work or made their problems worse, they could not get their money back. Good Feet said its "all sales are final" policy is posted in the stores.

That is unreasonable and just not fair! If someone's feet are hurting, do you think they are scanning the walls for a refund policy? I don't think so.

My favorite part of the segment takes place in the first 30 seconds when the owner of the arch support store is in the back room of her store. What you see are endless row after row of incredible overpriced, pre-made, arch supports. There is nothing custom-made about these arch supports. But there they are, lined up like toy soldiers by the thousands, waiting to make the storeowner a truckload of money!

Here is the link for the full news story from WISC-TV about "Good Feet" that you can watch.

> http://www.channel3000.com/video/4430559/detail.
> html

In Denver, KMGH-TV, the ABC affiliate, also ran a piece exposing "Good Feet" called:

> Do Good Feet's Claims Of Helping Foot
> Pain Stand? Doctors Say Sales People Can't
> Diagnose, Treat Problems

This story was great because the TV station used hidden cameras to go into various Good Feet stores in the greater Denver area, uncovering the truth about their operations. You can see this great segment at

> http://www.thedenverchannel.com/news/4979919/
> detail.html

Also from Denver, Craigslist went after Good Feet by putting up this link:

> http://denver.craigslist.org/for/827665253.html

Here is a story from Reno, Nevada that was on the web site www.Complaints.com, where the person's feet were made worse by Good Feet arch supports and they could not get a refund. The link is at

http://www.complaints.com/2006/december/29/Good_Feet_Store_10529.htm

And finally another unhappy Good Feet Customer spent almost $700 and their feet are worse, and of course, they could not get a refund. You can read this for yourself at

http://www.complaints.com/2007/april/9/GOOD_FEET_STORE_INSERTS_126347.htm

People are not only unhappy with "Good Feet's" sale practices. Here is a web site containing over 150 complaints/comments about Walkfit, a mail-order arch support.

http://www.infomercialscams.com/scams/walk_fit

Another chain of arch support stores called "The Ideal Feet Store" has also been beaten up on the internet for their sales practices.

The "Rip-Off Report," a very aggressive web site, started its attack on the Ideal Feet store of Plano TX, by printing what this unhappy customer wrote:

Beware of buying these orthotic/arch supports.

WARNING: The Ideal Feet Store sales people are con artists and will tell you anything to sell their arch support/orthotic devices at an outrageous price and there are NO REFUNDS or RETURNS. They are a Rip-Off! He goes on to say:

"I paid over $400.00 for crappy pieces of plastic to go into my shoes that caused physical health problems and these people couldn't care less! BUYER BEWARE."

This customer does not stop there. For the rest of his unhappy comments, go to

http://www.ripoffreport.com/reports/0/293/RipOff0 293423.htm

I saved the most important one for last. In another attack on the Ideal Feet Store posted on the "Rip-Off Report," a female customer from Tulsa, OK wrote:

I also purchased the Ideal Feet inserts and yes, I fell for all the foot print, hands in front and behind tests.

I spent $279.99 on original N11, $219.00 on Freedom 5, $19.99 on Cushion W10 and $110.00 on FRDM-Demo.

I have never been able to wear them as the pain is unreal. They just are not long enough from the ball of my foot to my heel.

There is a no exchange or refund clause on the sales ticket which I noticed after I was home.

I really don't see anything a person could do under these circumstances to get their money returned. I lost $629.97 + 8.52% in taxes.

To top things off, I went to the local dollar general and found the very same arch support for $8.00. I am serious! I bought a pair and brought them home. They are the exact same product, down to the vent holes. I repeat—nothing is different from the $8.00 pair and the $270.00 pair. Consumers please be aware!

Thank you ma'am. I am very sorry of your situation. You are the exact reason why I am writing this – to let people know about this rip off.

Equal Time

I am fully aware that there are alot of people satisfied with the arch supports or insoles that they bought from Good Feet, the Ideal Foot Store, or the trunk of some guy's car. I am very, very happy for you. That is great, but please allow me as a licensed foot specialist with a third of a century's experience to make you aware of the following points.

Regardless of whether you paid $19.95 or $699, you overpaid for these things by a lot. Don't believe me? Shop around and you can see for yourself. The same insoles you bought can be had for a fraction of the cost either at Wal-Mart, Target, Kmart or in catalogues. Trust me (I hope you do by now), there is no major difference. Just ask the nice lady above from Tulsa who went to the Dollar Store after spending almost $700.00 at Good Feet.

Even if you feel wonderful with your supports or insoles, you are not treating the real reason for your foot/arch pain. The problem is not your arch but the ball of your feet and the metatarsal bones. The Toe Pad or Shoe Insert, which cost three to four dollars, is far superior to any arch support bought at any price. The reason is simple. As I explained to you earlier in Chapters 3 and 4, the real reason for your foot problem is not your arch falling, but that you have a Morton's Toe. And it is the Morton's Toe that is causing your arch to fall. If you treat the Morton's Toe, your arch will not fall; hence, you will not need an overpriced arch support to start with. However, Dr. Dudley J. Morton, the leading medical expert on the human foot for the first half of the 20th Century, who taught at Yale and Columbia Medical Schools, and who wrote seven medical textbooks, might be wrong. And the nice person in the arch support store, who was selling double-wide mobile homes a week before you met, may be right. It really is a close call.

How many times in your life have you heard of a whole industry refusing to give a refund on their products? Heck, people can even return underwear and socks to some stores after wearing them for a month, and get their money back. (I swear!) What is so scary is that these arch support stores refuse to give any refunds! Is it because they know that if they gave refunds, their doors would not stay open for long? Gentlemen, if you want the authorities and me off of your back, start giving refunds like 99.99% of the rest of the civilized business world.

In my office, patients pay about $400 for custom-made orthotics. From what I can tell, this is a fair average of what most podiatrists charge for orthotics across the country. I only decide to make orthotics for a patient after I evaluate them and treat them for a while. Why do I wait, and not make it at once? The simple answer is that I am not sure orthotics will work for a patient until I see them several times and know they are going to work. You cannot determine if the patient will benefit from orthotics or even arch supports until you see how they are responding to treatment. Any good doctor will tell you the same. Besides, I am not going to ask someone to spend $400.00 of their money (or their insurance company's money) unless I truly believe it is going to work. After I take a custom cast (impression) of the feet, which then goes to a laboratory that specializes in making orthotics. It then takes several weeks for the orthotics to be fabricated. Once they arrive back from the laboratory the patient is fitted for them. Regardless of the reason, it the patient cannot get the orthotics to work to their satisfaction or is unhappy for any reason I will offer them a full refund. This has happened three times in the last five years. I cannot speak for every doctor but the ones I associate with would do the same exact thing.

In the end, there is no special shoe, good sneaker, right sandal, proper arch support, or exceptional insole for you. In the end, it all depends on the feet you were born with, and if they work correctly. Luckily for all us, even if they do not work correctly, we don't have to suffer. The proper treatment was developed by a physician born in the late 19th century in Baltimore with a funny first name.

APPENDIX

Glossary

Chapters 22 & 23 of Dr. Morton's
1935 book, The Human Foot
(compliments of Columbia University Press)

Dr. Morton's 1932 Patent

Glossary

Accommodate: to adapt, adjust or modify in order to help treat a condition. A Toe Pad accommodates the foot to work properly.

Addison's Disease: the chronic insufficiency of the hormone produced by the adrenal gland that results in bronzing of the skin, anemia, weakness, and low blood pressure.

Anatomical Position: the proper reference position when exact anatomic orientation is needed in performing some examination or task.

Bursa: a bursa is a sac filled with synovial fluid that acts as a shock absorber to reduce the stress between different tissues of the body.

Bursitis: an inflammation of a bursa.

Cartilage: the tissue that serves as the "cushion" between the bones of the joint. In most arthritis, it is the cartilage that wears down and causes pain.

Capsulitis: inflammation of the capsule, which is the tissue that acts as an envelope or surrounds the joint.

Colitis: Inflammation of the large intestine (the colon).

Compensate: to neutralize or counter balance, a defect, or unde-sired effects, of some abnormal condition. To compensate is not to cure but just to repair.

The Dudley J. Morton Foot (Long Second Metatarsal): term used by Dr. Janet Travell to denote a Morton's Toe.

Dog and Pony Show: any type of presentation or display that is somewhat contrived or overly involved in order to make the customer think they are buying a worthwhile produce or gadget. In advertising, the creative pitch is commonly referred to as the

"Dog and Pony" show.

ESPN: cable television network dedicated to broadcasting and producing sports-related programming 24 hours a day.

Fasciitis: see plantar fasciitis.

Gangrene: the death of tissue due to the loss of blood supply to that area, sometimes bacteria also invades accelerating the tissues decay. The two major types are gas gangrene and dry gangrene.

Hallux Abducto Valgus: a more complicated type of bunion deformity where the big toe is not only moving toward the 2nd toe, but where it may be over or under lapping the 2nd toe.

Inflammation: one of the basic way the body protects itself, when reaction to infection, irritation, or other injuries. It main features are redness, warmth, swelling and pain.

Joint: the place where two bones are attached for the purpose of motion. Their are different types of joints according to their motion: a ball and socket joint; a hinge joint; a condyloid joint; a pivot joint; gliding joint; and a saddle joint.

Lumbago: is the term used to describe general lower back pain involving the lumbar vertebrae.

Osteoarthritis: the most common form of arthritis caused by the wear and tear of the joint, resulting in the destruction of cartilage of the joint.

Periosteum: a thick covering of fibrous connective tissue that wraps itself around the bone. If torn it tends to bleed with the result of new bone being formed like in heel spurs.

Plantar Fasciitis: inflammation of the plantar fascia – the "bowstring-like" tissue stretching from the heel to the toes. It often appears with a heel spur.

Plantar Ligament: the tissue on the bottom of two bones, that binds them together.

Podiatrist: a physician and surgeon that specializes in the evaluation and treatment of diseases of the foot, ankle and leg.

Pronation: normal series of motions of the foot, where it becomes a bag of bones and less stable, so that it can meet the ground and accommodate to the new walking surface. It is the opposite of supination.

Referred Pain: Pain felt at a site other than where the cause is situated. This is a characteristic of Myofascial Pain Syndrome where pain in one spot will cause pain at a distal location.

Rigid Lever: This is what the foot must become during Supination in order for it to be stable so that it can push away from the ground. If the foot does not become the rigid lever at the proper time, it will over pronate causing most of the foot and body problems written about in this book. A Morton's Toe will intrinsically prevent the foot from becoming a rigid lever

Sciatic pain: also known as sciatica. Pain from inflammation or irritation of the sciatic nerve that can start in the low back and can go all the way down to the big toe.

Supination: normal series of motions of the foot, where it becomes a rigid lever and more stable, so it can support our body weight when it pushes off from the ground. It is the opposite of pronation.

Synovitis: an inflammation of the synovium.

Synovium: the lining of the joint. A layer of connective tissue that lines the inside of the joint, makes synovial fluid, which has a lubricating function.

Ulcer: an area of tissue erosion, that is always depressed below the level of the surrounding tissue.

XXII

SHORTNESS OF THE FIRST METATARSAL BONE

ONE of the requirements for ideal foot function is an equidistance of the heads of the first and the second metatarsal bones from the heel (fig. 78). Together the two form the fulcrum of the foot's leverage action; if they are not on a line with each other,

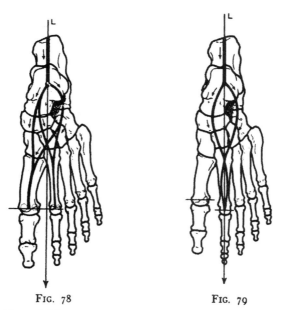

FIG. 78   FIG. 79

FIG. 78.—Normal Movement of Leverage Stresses on Each Side of the Leverage Axis, L

They converge on the bases of metatarsals I and II, being transmitted by these bones to the ground.

FIG. 79.—Leverage Stresses, Short First Metatarsal Bone

A short first metatarsal bone causes the second to act as the principal leverage member. The stresses converge upon the base of the latter only, being transmitted by it to the ground. Under the increased amount of function, metatarsal II becomes widened and hypertrophied; a correspondingly increased strain is imposed upon its basal joint.

the one fartherest forward will serve as the principal fulcrum and be subjected to a heavy concentration of functional stresses. Shortness of the first metatarsal bone as a cause of disorder is, therefore, associated essentially with locomotion and directly affects the fore part of the foot. It may also contribute to postural trouble, involving the longitudinal arch through a deficiency in medial support which this bone should normally furnish.

A comparison of Figures 78 and 79 demonstrates the difference in the movement of leverage stresses in the normal foot and in one of this type. In normal action, the medial and lateral lines of stress converge upon the bases of metatarsals I and II, whence they are transmitted to the ground by both bones. But with a short first metatarsal, since the head of the second occupies a more advanced position (and for this reason acts alone as the principal fulcrum of the foot), the medial and lateral lines of stress converge upon the base of the second metatarsal bone only, and then proceed to the ground through this bone. Continuation of their convergent movements from the two sides of the foot has the effect of widening its shaft, as shown in the illustration. In addition, the increased burden of body weight which this bone is forced to carry promotes a thickening of its cortical walls.

If we compare the vertical depth of the basal joint surfaces of metatarsals I and II (fig. 80), it will be observed that the first metatarsal bone is designed to withstand a load fully twice as heavy as the second metatarsal. In the condition under discussion, these burdens are reversed and the stresses of locomotion are at times intensified threefold or more upon the more weakly designed second metatarsal segment (including the middle cuneiform bone) and its joints. The enlargement of metatarsal II, previously described, implies compensatory changes in the plantar ligaments of the proximal joints also, so that under an ordinary range of function the foot may be protected sufficiently against harmful strain. But this improper distribution of stresses

SHORTNESS OF METATARSAL I   181

remains a potential source of trouble, and the joints are always susceptible to a tearing strain upon the plantar ligaments through some unusually strenuous physical effort. These two small joints, between the middle cuneiform and navicular bones posteriorly, and metatarsal II anteriorly, lie so deeply beneath the surface as to obscure the fact that here is the primary site of clinical symptoms, especially as the latter are usually manifested in a diffuse pain or discomfort which extends through the entire

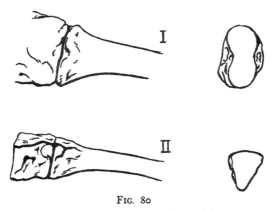

FIG. 80

Basal Joints of Metatarsals I and II

Lateral views of the first and second tarsometatarsal joints, and posterior (joint) surfaces of metatarsals I and II, showing the greater vertical depth and much stronger design of metatarsal I to resist vertical stresses.

fore part of the foot. Continued function during a period of acute strain leads very readily to a chronic traumatic arthritis in this part with more or less joint effusion, or synovitis. The thick and painful callosities which form in the middle of the ball of the foot are specific local reactions of the skin which are induced by the intense pressure caused by this concentration of weight. They develop under the head of the second, and sometimes of the third metatarsal bones.

The intense localized pressure which induces this growth of callus is a second direct cause of symptoms. Irritation of the cells of the basement membrane stimulates more rapid proliferation of the cells to form the callosities, and is accompanied by a burning sensation which results from irritation of peripheral nerve filaments. Later the growth of callus may become a new source of acute pain by acting as a foreign body. Thus callosities in this region are not to be regarded as mere incidental conditions, but as characteristic or keynote signs of abnormal foot function.

Shortness of the first metatarsal bone can hardly be called a definite abnormality. As indicated by these studies, it is of very common occurrence, and is transmitted in family strains (figs. 81, 82 A and B). Presumably it can be found in all races (figs. 83 and 84). Only under conditions of civilization, however, does a short first metatarsal bone become a positive factor tending toward clinical foot disorder. It rarely produces symptoms before adulthood, because during youth the general elasticity and resiliency of the tissues act automatically to modify any concentration of weight upon some single point in the foot's contact with the ground; but as the rigidity of matured tissues replaces their earlier elasticity, this self-adjusting quality becomes lost and the resulting concentration of stresses acquires harmful intensity.

Among men, feet with a short first metatarsal bone are not very frequently seen as clinical liabilities. The strains of ordinary function are probably taken care of because, the defect being congenital, compensatory strengthening of the tissues have been acquired during the periods of adolescence and early maturity. Nevertheless at any time a misstep, some strenuous sport, or unfavorable conditions of foot function may institute symptomatic disorder. Thus the male foot usually becomes affected only through some violent phase of locomotion activity, when the foot is being used as a lever.

Among women, however, the short first metatarsal bone is a common cause of pain and disability, through its association with the use of high-heeled shoes; for under these circumstances it affects the foot both in stance and in locomotion. In other

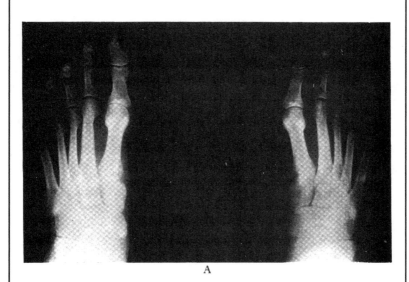

A

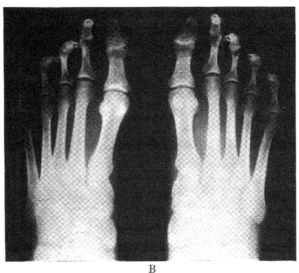

B

FIG. 81
Hereditary Transmission of Short First Metatarsal Bone
Instances of short first metatarsal bones in mother (A) and daughter, eighteen years (B). Note that the hypertrophy of metatarsal II is much greater in the older individual.

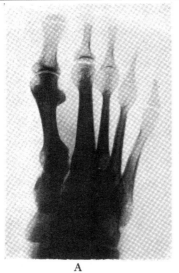
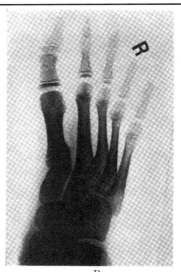

A   B

FIG. 82

Hereditary Transmission of Short First Metatarsal Bone

Similar evidence of congenital transmission of the short first metatarsal bone in mother (A) and daughter, nine years (B). In this instance even the hypertrophy of the second metatarsal bone appears to have attained an inheritable quality.

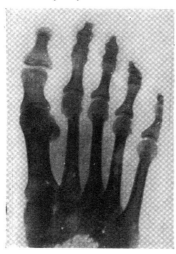
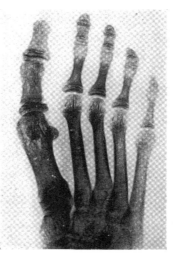

FIG. 83   FIG. 84

A Short First Metatarsal Bone A Short First Metatarsal Bone
in an African Native's Foot   in an African Native's Foot

Male, aged sixteen years   Female, aged fourteen years

SHORTNESS OF METATARSAL I 183

words, when the heel is raised to the height specified by designers of women's shoes, the foot is held in a *position of leverage,* and a short metatarsal I tends to lose its contact with the ground, so that body weight becomes concentrated upon the second metatarsal. The ensuing disorder is not a so-called "falling of the anterior metatarsal arch" as commonly understood, but an uneven distribution of weight upon the metatarsal bones whereby

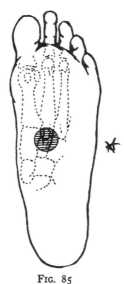

FIG. 85

Point of Metatarsal Tenderness

Plantar view of the foot showing the location of the typical point of deep tenderness over the basal joint of metatarsal II.

the artificially assumed "leverage" position of the foot in the presence of a short first metatarsal bone, causes the second to assume and to transmit the greater part of body weight.

As previously stated, the compensatory strengthening of metatarsal II and its basal joint begins apparently in childhood. As long as the stresses are kept within the margin of functional stimulation, this reinforcing growth progresses without clinical symptoms; but if the strain at any time exceeds that limit, a painful traumatic arthritis is started. A typical symptom appears as a result of such acute strain. It comprises a point of plantar tenderness located in this region and can be identified by deep pressure (fig. 85). At times the X-ray picture shows a sufficient degree of separation of the tarsal and metatarsal bones to indicate a definite synovitis of these midtarsal joints (see fig. 77).

Under continued trauma, cellular irritability extends to adjacent structures. Thus the close proximity of the Medial plantar nerve to the joint in question and the fanlike distribution of its branches through the metatarsal portion of the foot (fig. 86), explains the diffuse and indefinite pain experienced in the fore part of the foot. The pain is essentially a *referred* one, as the irritation is received apparently as the nerve trunk passes the joint. It varies greatly in intensity and may even be excruciating and shooting, corresponding to the metatarsalgia first described in 1875 by Professor T. G. Morton of the University of Pennsylvania.

External signs of a short first metatarsal bone are apparent but not conspicuous. The foot appears quite normal, and is usually well arched. Almost invariably the second toe is of greater length than the first. The dorsum of the foot immediately behind the toes, tends to present a roundness or convexity which is missing in an ideally designed foot. The presence of a callus under the head of metatarsal II is usually heavily developed in matured women of active habits; in younger or less active women, it may consist merely of a diffuse thickening of the skin which can be recognized only by comparing that area with the soft, thin skin beneath the head of metatarsal I. In men, owing to their use of low-heeled shoes, the formation of a callus in this region is much less, both in frequency and in amount.

The presence of painful callosities in the metatarsal region is conducive in time to the development of a general claw-toed deformity and, in the second digit, to the exaggerated distortion called "hammer-toe." Next to faulty footwear, uneven distribution of weight upon the metatarsal bones is the most frequent, and the most insidious cause of these toe deformities. The mechanism is easily understood. As painful callosites are developed, pressure upon them is subconsciously lessened by a hyperactivity of the Flexor digitorum longus muscle. Since its tendons pass immediately beneath the heads of the metatarsal bones, they are able by this stronger contraction to transfer a part of the pressure of body weight from the heads of the metatarsal bones directly forward upon the tips of the digits. At first the short plantar flexors are able to maintain the proximal phalanges of the digits in a normal position: but eventually, either because of the greater power of the long flexors, or because their lifting power is augmented as the tips of the digits are drawn back closer to the heads of the metatarsal bones, the toes gradually assume a "clawed" position where they subsequently become fixed by contractures. The proximal joints (metatarsophalangeal) are permanently hyperextended; the proximal interphalangeal joints are acutely flexed. The distal interphalangeal joints may be flexed or extended, the length of the digits being a determining factor. Short shoes or stockings hasten the deformity.

Posteriorly Located Sesamoid Bones

In a few cases observed in the original studies, a rearward position of the sesamoid bones, well toward the neck of the first metatarsal, was the most prominent of the three disturbing factors. These small bones are naturally mobile units because they are inclosed in the tendons of the two short flexors of the hallux (in association with the abductor and the adductor); but they move only as the proximal phalanx of the toes is flexed or extended. With the great toe in a middle, or neutral, position, one might expect the location of the sesamoids to be uniformly constant. X-ray pictures reveal, however, that this is not the case; the reason has not been determined. The effect of the position of the sesamoids upon the mechanism of the foot, however, is sufficiently apparent to merit consideration. Acting, as they do, as the bearing points of the first metatarsal bone, their position in relation to the head of metatarsal II influences the functional efficiency of these two bones. Their rearward position acts as a potential shortening of metatarsal I.

Thus, while posteriorly located sesamoid bones should be included as a recognizable factor in these disorders, until more information is gained it may be well to consider their part as contributory, rather than primarily causal.

XXIII

DORSAL HYPERMOBILITY OF THE FIRST METATARSAL SEGMENT

Of the three types of structural defects identified in these studies, hypermobility of the first metatarsal segment * is responsible for the widest range of foot trouble. It may be inherited or acquired

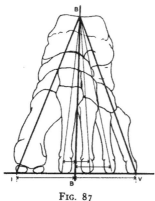

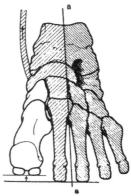

FIG. 87   FIG. 88

FIG. 87.—Structural Stability, Front View

Anterior view of the foot's framework with the axis of balance (BB) in normal position between metatarsals II and III. The first and fifth metatarsal bones furnish an equally wide margin of stability on each side of the foot (IB and BV).

FIG. 88.—Hypermobility of the First Metatarsal Segment

Foot skeleton with the first metatarsal and medial cuneiform bones unshaded, denoting their ineffectiveness (through hypermobility) to contribute to the medial stability of the foot. The resulting pronation causes body weight to become concentrated upon metatarsal II and continues until restricted by the muscles on the inner side of the ankle, or until metatarsal I gains a firm contact with the ground.

during early childhood. Laxity of the plantar ligaments of this segment affects both the longitudinal arch, by impairing the stability of the foot as a base of support, and the fore part of

* This refers to the first metatarsal and medial cuniform bones.

the foot, by causing an improper distribution of weight upon the metatarsal bones. The functional capabilities of these feet are lowered according to the degree of the abnormal mobility; if sufficiently great, only time and the continued use of the feet beyond their restricted capabilities is needed to produce serious disability and eventually a more or less complete breakdown of the entire foot structure. Comparison of Figures 87 and 88 shows how important is the part performed by the first metatarsal segment in furnishing medial stability to foot posture. For if through laxity of its plantar ligaments the weight-supporting effectiveness of the first metatarsal segment becomes lessened or lost, medial stability of the foot becomes reduced and dependent upon the second metatarsal segment, which remains as the only, and far less efficient, buttressing member of the inner side of the axis of balance.

As previously described in physiological studies, the significance of a pronated posture when the foot is bearing weight does not lie in the disalignment of the leg and foot, but in the abnormal position which the lower end of the tibia (representing the column of transmitted weight) occupies in relation to the area of ground contact. The location of the center of transmitted weight to the area of support determines not only the protective margins of security to foot balance, but also the ratio of weight distribution upon the different metatarsal segments. Any condition which disturbs those margins of structural stability and allows a corresponding shift in the weight center, will also cause an altered distribution of weight stresses through the entire foot. As a sign of disordered function, the faulty posture of pronation is useful in furnishing external evidence of a medial displacement of the weight center.

When normal effectiveness of the first metatarsal bone is reduced or eliminated through laxity of its plantar ligaments, the inner border of postural security becomes transferred to a line from the heel through metatarsal II (fig. 88). In addition, the double share of body weight normally borne by metatarsal I

HYPERMOBILITY OF METATARSAL I 189

falls upon the metatarsal II, tripling its burden. Unless the second metatarsal segment can withstand this overload, a stretching of its ligaments will allow the weight center to shift medially beyond its very limited margin of medial support, until its buttressing effect also will be eliminated.

At this point, one of two things will happen. If the hypermobility of metatarsal I has been slight, supporting contact of that bone is quickly made and further incursion of the weight

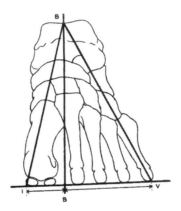

FIG. 89

First Degree Pronation, Front View

Altered position of the axis of balance (BB) in the first degree of pronation when it coincides with the leverage axis between metatarsals I and II. The foot still retains a serviceable margin of stability (IB) in spite of its reduced proportions to lateral stability (BV).

center is arrested before it has passed to the medial side of the leverage axis. The first metatarsal bone thus regains its function with a mild degree of pronation, but stands alone as the single buttress against further inward displacement of the weight center. The latter is now maintained in a vertical plane coinciding with the leverage axis, instead of in the normal plane of balance (figs. 89, 90 P). This represents what is commonly regarded as the first degree of pronation. Such feet are quite capable and efficient; the fact that they are often observed in runners and sprinters testifies to their functional capabilities, at least, in locomotion. Also, X-ray evidence of such hypermobility is found in the feet of African natives, who are notably free of any symptomatic disorder (figs. 91, 92). The single intimation that such feet are not as strong as the ideal structure lies in the fact that they tire more easily under prolonged standing. This is explained

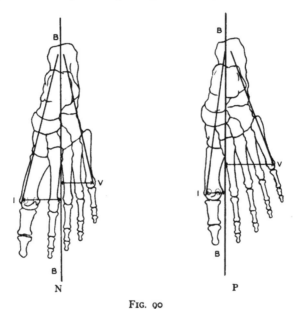

FIG. 90

Structural Stability, Normal and First Degree Pronation

Top view of normal (N) and first degree pronated (P) feet, showing the difference in the inner and outer margins of stability.

by the fact that even this mild degree of pronation is associated with some increase of weight distribution upon the medial segments of the foot.

However, if the laxity of the plantar ligaments of the first metatarsal segment is greater than in the condition just described, and if a supporting contact with the ground is not made, then the disordered phases of function become more complex and extensive.

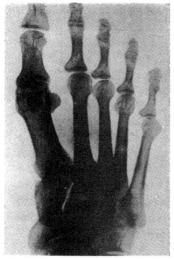 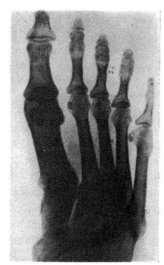

Fig. 91   Fig. 92

Fig. 91.—Evidence of Hypermobility of the First Metatarsal Segment
in an African Native Aged Sixty Years

Hypertrophy of metatarsal II can be noted. also the separation between
the medial and the middle cuneiform bones.

Fig. 92.—Hypermobility of the First Metatarsal Segment in an African
Native Aged Twenty Years

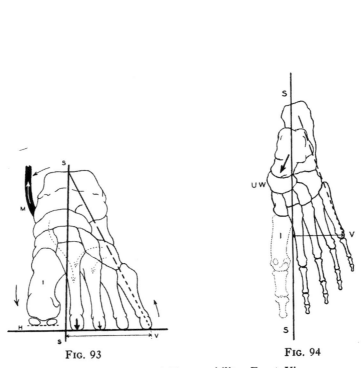

FIG. 93   FIG. 94

FIG. 93.—Advanced Degree of Hypermobility, Front View

Medial unbalance of the foot beyond first degree of pronation, owing to hypermobility of the first metatarsal segment indicated at H. As the foot rolls inward, the outer border tends to be lifted from the ground, eliminating active support by the outer metatarsals and concentrating weight on metatarsal II as indicated by the short heavy arrows. The dotted arrows show the direction of weight stresses. The previous axis of balance is now a single line of structural support (SS). There is no margin of medial stability to the inner side of the line SS. The foot rolls inward until arrested by the supinating muscles (M) or by the ultimate contact of metatarsal I with the ground.

FIG. 94.—Advanced Degree of Hypermobility, Top View

The ineffectiveness of the first metatarsal bone due to laxity of its plantar ligaments is suggested by its dotted outline. The arrow indicates the inward deflection of unbalanced body weight (UW) off the inner border of the foot. Inward rotation of the talus is indicated by the medial prominence of the navicular bone.

HYPERMOBILITY OF METATARSAL I   191

(1) Under the triple load imposed on metatarsal II, its plantar ligaments are strained and its tarsal joints become chronically traumatized even under the stresses of ordinary function. (2) With stretching of the ligaments and loss of the narrow buttressing margin afforded by metatarsal II, the inward movement of the weight center continues until stopped by the action of the supinating muscles (particularly the Tibialis posterior and the Flexor digitorum longus), or until the first metatarsal segment acquires a later firm contact with the ground (figs. 93, 94). As a matter of fact, both conditions occur in varying degree. For, following a period of rest, the muscles will usually accept the burden of displaced weight in order to sustain the posture of the foot as nearly normal as possible; but after being subjected to this abnormal phase of function for a time, they tire and allow the foot to sag inwardly until the first metatarsal segment acquires its contact and relieves them of the load. (3) The inward roll of the foot increases the obliquity of the sustentaculum tali, which supports the head of the talus. Then, as in the prehuman foot, this obliquity causes body weight to be more strongly deflected toward the medial border (fig. 94). In addition, it influences the anteroposterior axis of the talus to rotate inwardly. This means that owing to the mortiselike articulation of the talus with the leg bones, the leg is also rotated inwardly. Consequently, the forward movement of the leg upon the foot in locomotion is performed at an angle with the inner border of the latter instead of coinciding with its longitudinal axis. A compensatory external rotation at the hip joint to correct this internal rotation of the leg, gives the foot an increased out-toed posture and emphasizes more strikingly the abducted position of the fore part of the foot as a secondary structural deformity. (4) With the loss of foot balance, the outer border tends to roll upward. Thus the lateral metatarsal bones lose their firm supporting contact and the weight normally distributed to them is added to the burden concentrated upon metatarsal II. (5) These faulty changes in the foot's mechanism create abnormal strains upon

the muscles and the ligaments on the medial side of the ankle and the foot. Also the distorted movements of gravitational and propulsive stresses combined with spasm of the peroneal muscles, cause the midtarsal bones to be forced into twisted and uneven contacts with each other (fig. 95). Under such pressure the shapes of these bones become so altered that their original alignment is destroyed as may be observed in an angulation between the axes of the tarsal and the metatarsal units (fig. 96). This

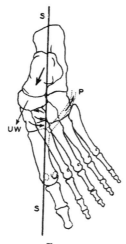

FIG. 95

Faulty Movements of Stresses

An exaggerated position of pronation showing the movement of unbalanced weight (UW) off the inner border of the foot and the opposing pull of peroneal spasm (P) across the instep. The small arrows indicate the distorting twist of these forces upon the tarsal bones, causing uneven contacts which result in the typical deformity shown in Fig. 96. Note the abduction of the fore part of the foot in relation to the posterior half.

distortion of their normal alignment comprises the structural changes by which the foot becomes flattened and loses its effectiveness as a lever. Its relation to the peroneal pull is easily discernible.

In applying this analysis of the disordered mechanism to clinical manifestations, two sites can be recognized as the sources

HYPERMOBILITY OF METATARSAL I   193

from which the original onset of symptoms develop: (1) the basal joints of the second metatarsal segment due to its heavily increased burden; and (2) the supinating muscles of the ankle which become strained and exhausted in their attempt to maintain balance in a structurally unstable foot.

The early symptoms may appear in either or both of these sites. If the greater amount of functional strain is received upon the basal joints of metatarsal II, then the symptoms are typically metatarsalgic in character. If, on the other hand, the activities of the individual are such as to place the greater strain upon the muscles, tiredness and aching of those tissues will be the prominent symptom, often associated with spasms at night.

As the disorder progresses, strain of the ligaments on the medial side of the ankle and foot is manifested by soreness and points of tenderness, until the entire arch of the foot may become extremely painful. During the early stage of strain, although the pain is diffuse and promotes the impression that the entire foot is breaking down, the trouble is definitely centered about the middle cuneiform bone as a focal point; for not only is this bone directly involved with metatarsal II in the concentration of weight stresses, but it also occupies the very center of distorted movements of force, which squeeze it into uneven contact with all of the adjacent bones. A local traumatic synovitis is inevitable. Inflammatory effusion tends to separate the joint surfaces and to permit minor painful movements or displacements between the bones. A symptom particularly suggestive of this synovitis is shown in patients who suffer severe pain when first putting their weight on their feet after an interval of rest, or upon arising; quite characteristically, this severe pain subsides soon after the bones have become adjusted under the assumption of weight.

More or less extensive nerve disorders develop in the persistently acute, or long-continued subacute cases. Motor, sensory and vasomotor nerves are all involved to a varying degree. Irritability of the motor nerves is manifested first in muscle spasm and during later stages by more or less interference in the coördination of locomotor movements. The scope of sensory disturbances is quite wide; it includes various types of pain ranging from a dull aching discomfort to pain of excruciating acuteness; also referred pains may extend downward to the toes or up to the legs and thighs to the back; local areas of tenderness, numbness or tingling are manifestations of sensory disturbances. The vasomotor disturbances are indicated by general sluggishness in the vascular circulation of the feet, and include symptoms of sweating, edema, pallor and mottled discoloration. The scope of these symptoms demonstrates the extent to which continued traumatic irritation disrupts the entire local nervous organization.

These nerve manifestations comprise, of course, the most conspicuous range of clinical symptoms, both subjective and objective. They are not the disorder itself, but the vehicle by which the degree of internal traumatism is revealed, and they form the usual criterion by which the clinical condition is differentiated from the preclinical.

In summarizing, it may be stated that hypermobility of the first metatarsal segment is a common cause of disordered function, and consequently, of reduced physical capabilities. If the individual, through disposition or circumstances, does not extend his physical activities beyond his restricted margin of safety, he will never become a clinical case, even though the structural fault within his feet is so great as to cause a serious disorder in their mechanism. On the other hand, this type of defect is capable of extensive disabling and deforming changes throughout the feet, if their restricted powers are habitually transgressed. The stresses of function are intensified upon the units of the second metatarsal segment. Here traumatic cellulitis results, in accordance with the intensity and duration of the strain. Involvement of adjacent tissues naturally includes the nerves, first in the form of a congestive irritability and later, as traumatic neuritis. The subjective symptoms now appear and are to be regarded as an index to the inflammatory state of the internal parts. Distortion

HYPERMOBILITY OF METATARSAL I   195

of the midtarsal bones under their uneven contacts, shown in Figure 96, is undoubtedly hastened by some degree of inflammatory softening. With the advance in bony changes, the leverage ability of the foot becomes permanently lost and locomotion is performed with the awkward gait of the "heel-walker."

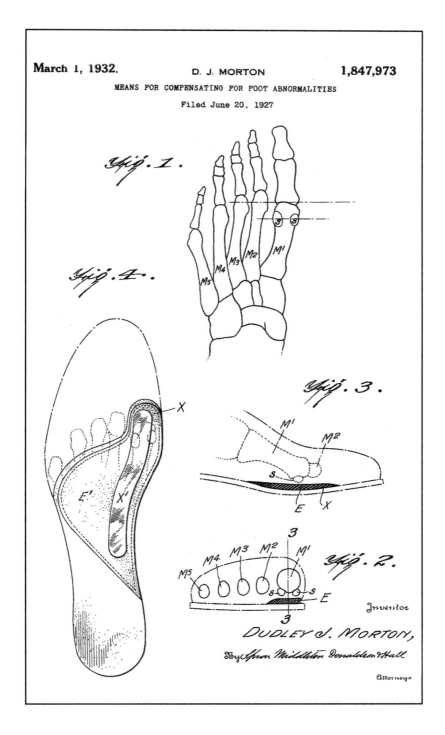

Patented Mar. 1, 1932

1,847,973

UNITED STATES PATENT OFFICE

DUDLEY J. MORTON, OF NEW HAVEN, CONNECTICUT

MEANS FOR COMPENSATING FOR FOOT ABNORMALITIES

Application filed June 20, 1927. Serial No. 199,953.

In the course of my investigations concerning the human foot, I have discovered that in some individuals there is an undue shortness of the first metatarsal bone, so that it does not extend as far forward as the second, or in some cases even the third. As a result, the longer metatarsal bones receive the concentrated stresses of body weight in walking and in other locomotor activities, while the first metatarsal bone fails to perform its proper share of function. Such unequal distribution of functional stresses is a frequent cause of severe pain and discomfort in the forepart of the foot, and of painful callosities.

In some other feet, I have found that the anterior ends (heads) of the first and second metatarsal bones are on a line with each other, being equi-distant from the heel, but the sesamoid bones which represent the point of ground contact of the first metatarsal bone, are located rearwardly relative to the head of the second metatarsal bone. The effect upon the foot's function is similar to that produced by a short first metatarsal bone.

The present invention aims to provide a method of and means for compensating for such morphologic variations and avoiding or removing the pain and discomfort not infrequently attendant therewith, and the invention includes the novel method and means hereinafter described and defined in the appended claims.

In order that the invention may be more readily understood reference is made to the accompanying drawings, in which:—

Figure 1 is a plan view of the bones of the forward portion of a human foot having such comparatively short first metatarsal bone.

Fig. 2 is a cross section through a shoe (shown conventionally) to illustrate my method and means for correcting the effects of the abnormal condition, the bones being shown in their relative positions, but all else omitted.

Fig. 3 is a section on line 3—3 of Fig. 2, with the relative position of the head of the second metatarsal bone indicated, and

Fig. 4 is a diagrammatic plan view illustrating a modification.

In Figure 1 which is a reproduction from an X-ray photograph of such a type of foot, the metatarsal bones are designated respectively M1, M2, M3, M4 and M5 and it will be observed that the first bone M1 is considerably shorter than the second M2 or even the third M3, and such a condition under locomotor activities the pain and other troubles hereinbefore referred to.

I have discovered that by placing beneath that portion of the foot which underlies the front end of the first metatarsal bone a thickness of supporting material, such as indicated at E, this will compensate for its relative shortness in stance and make the foot function in locomotor activities, like an ordinary foot, thereby avoiding the distressing results which usually follow such a structural variation.

The same thing is true in cases where the ends of the first and second metatarsal bones are in line, but the sesamoid bones (indicated at s s in the same figures for convenience) are located rearwardly relative to the head of the second metatarsal bone.

The essential features of the present invention are; (1) providing a sufficient difference in thickness of material (E) interposed between the foot and the supporting surface or ground, beneath the head of the first metatarsal bone on the one hand, and the adjacent metatarsal bones on the other, the greater thickness underlying the first metatarsal in order to compensate for its relative shortness in stance; and (2) a forward extension of the material E (as X in Fig. 3) beyond the line of the basal joint of the great toe in order to make it effective as an artificial extension of the first metatarsal bone in the leverage action of the foot. Although distinctly different in their fundamental action, these two features or elements are intimately related because they apply to the two phases of foot function; either of them may be employed separately, but they are preferably and more properly used in combination.

The increased thickness of material (E) underlying the ball of the great toe may be

2   1,847,973

designated a "metatarsal lift". If carried beyond the forward end of the first metatarsal bone as X, it is ordinarily effectual as an artificial extension of that bone, because the greater depth of material furnishes some degree of increased rigidity in that area. A more rigid extension X 1 (Fig. 4) however, may comprise a strip or plate of metal or other suitable material, which extends from some rearward position to beyond the head of the first metatarsal bone and under the base of the great toe. Also, such an extension may be incorporated in the design of an arch support or other device, as a supplementary feature; the present models of arch support extending practically to, but not beyond, the head of the first metatarsal bone.

It is not an uncommon procedure in the treatment of pronation (commonly termed "weak ankles", "fallen arches") to supplement a wedge on the inner side of the heel of a shoe, with another wedge along the inner border of the sole. In pronation the inward roll of the ankle causes a concentration of body weight upon the inner arched border of the foot; consequently these combined wedges are used in order to more effectively tilt the foot outwardly and thereby transpose the concentration of body weight toward the outer border of the foot. Such a combination of wedges produces an absolutely different effect than is indicated or desired in the present case. In a foot with a short first metatarsal bone, the object to be accomplished is to elevate the supporting surface beneath the head of the first metatarsal, and to extend its effective leverage action so that this bone will be caused to assume a greater share of functional stresses, and in doing so, to relieve the second metatarsal from an undue concentration of such stresses, without the mechanism of the entire foot being disturbed or altered.

These features may be applied directly in the making of a shoe, or by subsequent alterations, in two ways: (1) by reducing the material of the sole which lies under the second and third metatarsals, or (2) by the insertion of extra material to underlie the first metatarsal bone. As another mode of application, the features may be incorporated in an insole or some other foot device, to be worn within the shoe. (Fig. 4.)

When using the device in the form of a removable insole, the added thickness of material (E') may be extended backwardly to stiffen the middle section of the insole against wrinkling, and laterally so that padding of some sort can be held in the area behind the heads of the second and third metatarsals, to further reduce the pressure exerted at the points of their ground contact where painful callosities have been formed in a large per cent of such cases.

It will be understood that when I use the term "article of footwear" herein it is intended in the broad sense and to be inclusive of not only shoes of all kinds, but insoles, devices, or attachments to be used with shoes.

What is claimed is:

1. A device adapted to be worn under the foot in a shoe, comprising a flat piece of leather or other suitable material, which extends from beneath the heel, forwardly to a transverse line immediately behind the heads of the four outer metatarsal bones, and with an extension which continues forward beneath the head of the first metatarsal bone.

2. A device of the nature of an insole, extending from under the heel, forwardly to a line immediately behind the heads of the four outer metatarsal bones, and having an extension which continues forwardly beneath the head of the first metatarsal bone, this extension being of greater thickness than the main portion of the insole.

3. A device of the nature of an insole extending from a rearward position, from under the heel, forwardly to a transverse line close behind the heads of the four outer metatarsal bones, and continuing forwardly beneath the head of the first metatarsal bone, the said device being two-layered or split, and suitably joined so as to allow for adjustment of thickness in the extended area and in the central portion behind the metatarsal heads by means of various thicknesses of inserts.

4. An insole extending from under the heel forwardly to a line closely behind the heads of the four outer metatarsal bones, and continuing forwardly beneath and beyond the head of the first metatarsal bone, and having a relatively rigid strip or plate positioned along and under the inner border of said insole and continuing forwardly beneath its extended portion underlying the base of the great toe.

5. The combination with a shoe sole of an inner member carried thereby and lying beneath and corresponding substantially in width to the head of the first metatarsal bone of the wearer and supporting said first metatarsal bone upon a relatively horizontal plane abruptly raised above the surface which supports the heads of the four outer metatarsal bones.

6. The combination with a shoe sole of an inner member overlying the shank thereof having the major portion of its forward edge located on a line immediately behind the location of the heads of the four outer metatarsal bones and with the remaining portion provided with an extension continuing forward beneath the location of the head of the first metatarsal bone.

7. A shoe having a sole provided on its upper face with a raised portion positioned to underlie the head of the first metatarsal bone and being of substantially the same width as said bone, said raised portion being

1,847,973   **3**

of uniform thickness in transverse section
and tapering towards the front and back of
the shoe.

8. A shoe having a sole provided on its
5 upper face with a raised portion positioned
to underlie the head of the first metatarsal
bone and being of substantially the same
width as said bone, said raised portion being
of uniform thickness in transverse section
10 and tapering towards the front and back of
the shoe and having its longitudinal edge
adjacent the outer side of the shoe inclined.

In testimony whereof, I affix my signature.
DUDLEY J. MORTON.

15

20

25

30

35

40

45

50

55

BIBLIOGRAPHY

NOTES

INDEX

Bibliography

Cailliet, Rene. *Foot and Ankle Pain.* Philadelphia: F.A. Davis, 1968.

Dallek, Robert. *An Unfinished Life: John F. Kennedy.* Boston: Little Brown, 2003.

Inman, Verne. *Durvries' Surgery of the Foot.* Third edition, Saint Louis: The C.V. Mosby Company, 1973.

Morton, Dudley J. Metatarsus Atavicus: The Identification of a Distinctive Type of Foot Disorder. *J. Bone Joint Surg. Am.,* 9: 531-544. 1927.

Morton, Dudley J. Hypermobility of The First Metatarsal Bone: The Interlinking Factor Between Metatarsalgia and Longitudinal Arch Strains, *J. Bone Joint Surg. Am.,* 10: 187 – 196, 1928.

Morton, Dudley J. Structural Factors in Static Disorders of the Human Foot. *Am J Surgery* 9: 315-326., 1930.

Morton, Dudley J. *The Human Foot, its evolution, physiology and functional disorder.* Columbia University Press, New York: 1935. Reprinted 1964 Hafner Publishing Co.

Morton, Dudley J. *Oh, Doctor! My Feet!,* New York: Appleton-Century Company, 1939.

Morton, Dudley J. *Human Locomotion and Body Form; a Study of Gravity and Man.* (with Dudley Dean Fuller) Baltimore: The Williams & Wilkins Company, 1952. Published overseas by Bailliere, Tindall, and Cox Ltd, London: 1952.

Rachlin, Edward. *Myofascial Pain and Fibromyalgia.* St Louis: The Mosby Company, 1994.

Schuler, Burton. *The Agony of De-Feet: a podiatrist guide to foot care.* The La Luz Press, 1982.

Travell, Janet G., Simons, David. *Myofascial Pain & Dysfunction: The Trigger Point Manual.* Baltimore: Williams & Wilkins, Volume 1 (1983), Volume 2 (1992)

Travell, Janet G. *Office Hours: Day and Night.* The World Publishing Company, New York: 1968.

Notes

Abbreviations

HF   Morton, Dudley J. *The Human Foot, its evolution, physiology and functional disorder.* New York: Columbia University Press, 1935.

MET Morton, Dudley J. Metatarsus Atavicus: The Identification Of A Distinctive Type Of Foot Disorder, *J. Bone Joint Surg. Am* 9: 531–544, 1927.

MYO Travell, Janet G., Simons, David. *Myofascial Pain & Dysfunction: The Trigger Point Manual,* Baltimore: Williams & Wilkins, Volume 1 (1983), Volume 2 (1992).

HL   Morton, Dudley J., Fuller, Dudley D. *Human Locomotion and Body Form; a Study of Gravity and Man,* Baltimore: Williams & Wilkins, 1952.

FB   Rachlin, Edward. *Myofascial Pain and Fibromyalgia,* St. Louis: The Mosby Company, 1994.

OFF Travell, Janet G. *Office Hours: Day and Night,* the World Publishing Company, New York: 1968.

Chapter 1: The Best $8.00 I Ever Spent

1. HF.
2. MET.
3. ibid.
4. OFF.
5. Note dated June 23, 1961 from Robert F. Kennedy to George McGovern. John F. Kennedy Presidential Library and Museum, Research Room, Robert F. Kennedy's papers, Attorney General's Papers, Personal Correspondence, Maas-Metropolitan", Box 2.
6. MYO.
7. Travell, Janet G. *The Dudley Morton Foot,* (Video), Baltimore: Williams & Wilkins, 1990.
8. Schuler, Burton. *The Agony of De-Feet: a podiatrist guide to foot care,* The La Luz Press, 1982.

Chapter 2: What is a Morton's Toe?

1. MYO p. 381.
2. HF p. 151.
3. HL pp. 121-125.
4. MYO.
5. MET.

Chapter 3: Do You Have a Morton's Toe, or the Wrong Type of Inheritances?

1. Schuler, Burton. *The Agony of De-Feet: a podiatrist guide to foot care,* The La Luz Press, 1982. p. 65
2. HL p. 118.
3. HF p. 182.
4. ibid. pp. 180-185.
5. ibid.
6. ibid. 179-186.
7. ibid. pages 187-195.
8. ibid. p 187.
9. ibid.
10. ibid. p. 187-188.

Chapter 4: Pronation, Morton's Toe, and How the Foot Works

1.   HL p. 122.

Chapter 5: Condition of the Foot Caused by Morton's Toe

1.   HF p. 193.

2.   Morton, Dudley J. *Hypermobility of the First Metatarsal Bone: The Interlinking Factor between Metatarsalgia and Longitudinal Arch Strains* (J. Bone Joint Surg. Am., 10: 187 – 196, 1928.

3.   HF.

4.   Morton, Dudley J. *Oh, Doctor! My Feet!* New York and London: Appleton-Century Company, Incorporated, 1939.

5.   HL.

6.   HF p. 193.

7.   ibid.

8.   ibid.

9.   Morton, Thomas G. A Peculiar and Painful Affection of the Fourth Metatarsophalangeal Articulation. *Am. J. Med. Sc.* LXXI, 37, 1876.

10. Schuler, Burton. *The Agony of De-Feet: a podiatrist guide to foot care,* The La Luz Press, 1982. pp. 123-124.

11. MET.

12. HF.

13. Morton, Thomas G. Peculiar and Painful Affection of the Fourth Metatarsophalangeal Articulation. *Am. J. Med. Sc.* LXXI, 37, 1876.

14. MET.

15. Morton, Thomas G. The Application of the X-rays to the Diagnosis of Morton's Painful Affection of the Foot or Metatarsalgia. *International Med. Mag.* V, 322, 1896.

16. ibid.

17. MET.

18. HF.

19. American Arthritis Foundation Web site.

20. FDS News, FDA Orders Unapproved Quinine Drugs from the Market and Cautions Consumers About "Off-Label" Use of Quinine to Treat Leg Cramps, December 11, 2006.

21. HF p. 193.

22. Restless Legs Syndrome Foundation, www.rls.org.

23. ibid.

24. *New York Times,* November 5, 1935.

25. *Banged Up and Bruised Boomers Weekend Warriors,* By Daryn Eller Web MD Feature.

Chapter 7: Myofascial Pain Syndrome, Morton's Toe, and Why You Can Really Hurt All Over

1. MYO.

2. ibid. Vol. I Chapter 4.

3. ibid.

4. OFF pp. 301-302.

5. ibid. p. 302.

6. ibid. p. 301.

7. MYO Vol. II p. 150.

8. ibid. pp. 168- 169.

9. FB pp. 229.

10. MYO p. 250.

11. ibid. p. 370.

12. ibid. p. 461.

13. ibid. p. 487.

14. Travell, J.G.; *The Dudley Morton Foot,* Video, Williams & Wilkins, Baltimore: 1990.

15. FB.

16. Dunteman Edwin. *Fibromyalgia and Myofascial Pain Syndromes, Practical Pain Management,* July/August 2004, Volume 4, Issue 4, pp. 26-29.

Chapter 8: The Toe Pad and Other Treatments for Morton's Toe

1. U.S. Patent # 1,847,973, of March 1, 1932.

2. MYO p. 390.

3. HF p. 220.

4. ibid. p. 221.

5. ibid.

Chapter 10: Dr. Dudley Joy Morton

1. Oh Doctor, My Feet! *The Readers Digest,* April 1939. pp. 95-98.

2. *Time Magazine,* April 12, 1926.

3. *New York Times,* August 16, 1922.

4. DUDLEY MORTON, SURGEON, 76, DIES, *New York Times,* May 23, 1960.

5. Morton Dudley J. *Grampa's Toy Shop,* Grampa Co. 1922.

6. MET.

7. Morton, Dudley J. Hypermobility of the First Metatarsal Bone: The Interlinking Factor between Metatarsalgia and Longitudinal Arch Strains, *J. Bone Joint Surg. Am.,* 10: 187-196, 1928.

8. Oh Doctor, My Feet! *The Readers Digest,* April 1939. pp. 95-98.

9. "Boy Meets Girl Meets Foot" *The New Yorker Magazine,* May 1939.

10. SCIENCE IN THE NEWS, Finding Out Why Feet Ache. *New York Times,* January 18, 1942.

11. Something Wrong with Your Feet, *The Reader's Digest,* December 1949.

12. HL.

13. Published overseas by Bailliere, Tindall, and Cox Ltd, London: 1952.

14. Personal Communication with Christopher Morton, February 2007.

15. Personal Communication with Alexander Morton, February 2007.

16. DUDLEY MORTON, SURGEON, 76, DIES, *New York Times,* May 23, 1960.

Chapter 11: Janet Travell, M.D.

1. The Janet G. Travell M.D. Papers, The George Washington University, The Melvin Gelman Library.

2. OFF p. 131.

3. Ibid. p. 252.

4. Travell J, Rinzler SH, Pain and Disability of the Shoulder and Arm. Treatments by Intramuscular Infiltration with Procaine Hydrochloride *Journal of the American Medical Association,* CXX, 1942. pp. 417-22

5. Travell J, Rinzler SH. The Myofascial Genesis of Pain. *Postgraduate Medicine* (1952); 11:425-34

6. Obituary, *New York Times,* August 3, 1997.

7. OFF pp. 5-6.

8. ibid.

9. ibid.

10. Dallek, Robert, *An Unfinished Life: John F. Kennedy 1917-1963* Boston: Little Brown and Company, 2003. pp. 34-37, 73-78.

11. ibid.

12. ibid. pp. 100-102.

13. ibid. p. 105.

14. ibid. p. 196.

15. ibid. p. 212.

16. OFF p. 330.

17. John F. Kennedy Presidential Library and Museum, Research Room, Robert F. Kennedy's papers, Attorney General's Papers, Personal Correspondence, Maas-Metropolitan", Box 2.

18. Pioneering Physician, Janet Grame Travell, *New York Times,* January 27, 1961.

19. Obituary, *New York Times*, August 3, 1997.

20. *New York Times,* June 14, 1961.

21. OFF p. 6.

22. ibid. p. 7.

23. Obituary, *New York Times,* August 3, 1997.

24. OFF.

25. MYO.

Chapter 12: More About Myofascial Pain and Morton's Toe

1. MYO Vol. I p. 112.

2. Ibid. p. 227.

3. Ibid. p. 166.

4. Phone conversation with David Simons, M.D. June 12, 2007.

5. FB p. 1.

6. Ibid. p. 17.

7. OFF pp. 261-262.

8. FB p. 412.

9. ibid. p. 41.

Chapter 13: Diabetic Ulcers, Amputations and the Morton's Toe

1. National Center for Chronic Disease Prevention and Health Promotion, National Estimates on Diabetes, December 20, 2005.

2. American Academy of Wound Management.

Chapter 14: More About Dudley Joy Morton, M.D.

1. *New York Times,* April 16, 1922.

2. *Albuquerque Journal,* March 16, 1935.

3. *New York Times,* February 26, 1939.

4. "Boy Meets Girl Meets Foot" *The New Yorker Magazine,* May 13, 1939.

5. "Boy Meets Girl Meets Foot", *Most of the Most of S.J. Pearlman,* Modern Library, 2000.

6. *Time Magazine,* January 26, 1942.

7. *New York Times,* January 18, 1942.

8. HL.

Chapter 15: Arch Supports and the Scam that Goes with Them

1. *New York Times,* January 18, 1942.

2. *Time Magazine,* January 24, 1942.

Index